THE ULTIMATE BBQ BOOK FOR MEN

101 Things Every Barbecue Lover Should Know

JACK ROSS

FREE BONUS

SCAN TO GET OUR NEXT BOOK FOR FREE!

TABLE OF CONTENTS

INTRODUCTION

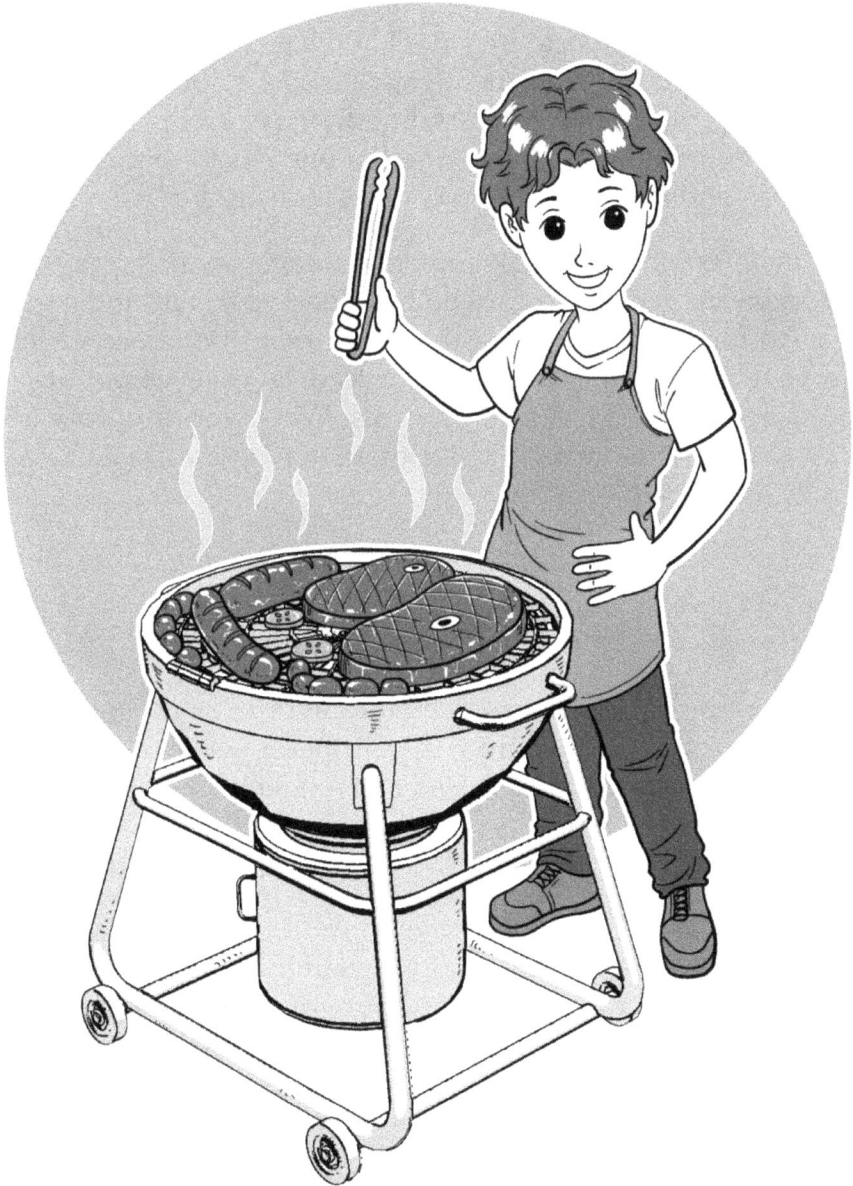

WELCOME TO THE WORLD OF BBQ

Barbecue is more than just a way of cooking; it's a phenomenon. If you've ever stood in front of the grill, tongs in one hand and a beer in the other, with the steaming scent of meat sizzling over an open flame filling your nose, then you already know. BBQ is the consummate man's pastime: bonding with friends, mastering fire like a caveman king, and enjoying life one smoky bite at a time. Fire, meat, and beer... What more can a man ask for?

BBQ involves much more than merely tossing some burgers onto your backyard grill. It requires both patience and skill, and it's also a way to form connections with others. From the dawn of time, men have circled flames not just to feed themselves but also to share stories, jokes, and achievements. When you fire up a BBQ today, you're reliving that history by keeping the flame alive—literally and metaphorically.

A SHORT HISTORY OF BBQ

The history of BBQ is just as rich and flavorful as the food itself. The word *barbecue* derives from the Caribbean word for this slow-cooking technique, *barbacoa*, based on wooden racks situated over a fire. Explorers took the art of barbacoa from the Caribbean, and as it spread around the world, different cultures adapted it in various ways.

Over the years, BBQ became a social event in the American South, with entire hogs consumed after hours of slow smoking. These traditions live on today. The Argentinian custom of *asado* involves cooking an entire meal over an open flame. In Korea, friends sizzle marinated meats over flames situated on the tabletop as they eat. Whether it's everyday BBQ from Texas or the flavorful profile of jerk chicken from Jamaica, BBQ is an endless form of expression. Yet all share the same heartbeat: fire, smoke, and camaraderie.

2

HOW TO USE
THIS BOOK

This book contains 101 tips, traits, techniques, and ideas any good BBQ man should know. You can read through chapter by chapter or skip around by jumping right to what you need in the moment. The choice is yours.

Interested in learning about charcoal versus gas grills? Start with the first chapter. Want to learn how to make dry rubs or sauces, or level up your spice game? Head to chapter four. Wondering about the best way to smoke a brisket or rack of ribs like professionals? Check out chapter six. No matter how you read it, consider this your BBQ playbook. Each section is full of useful tips and tricks, easy recipes, and enough humor to keep it enjoyable.

A WORD ABOUT
SAFETY

Before you toss steaks on the fire, let's make one thing clear: BBQ is serious business. Fire, sharp knives, and raw meat require respect. Please take safety seriously.

Keep a fire extinguisher nearby just in case. Wash your hands, tools, and surfaces religiously so that you don't send anyone to the hospital with food poisoning. Follow the temperature guides on cooking meat through. And please, for your dignity and your guests' health, do *not* soak your grill with lighter fluid like it's perfume!

BBQ should be about good food and a good time, not an ER visit. Respect for fire and food will gain you the respect of everyone around the table.

LET'S START SMOKING

Now that we've gotten the formalities out of the way, let's get to it. Whether this is your first BBQ or you're an experienced pitmaster looking to improve, this book will help you understand better flavor, make fewer mistakes, and hold hotter cookouts. So grab a cold beer, roll up your sleeves, and let's get cooking!

CHAPTER ONE:
BBQ FUNDAMENTALS

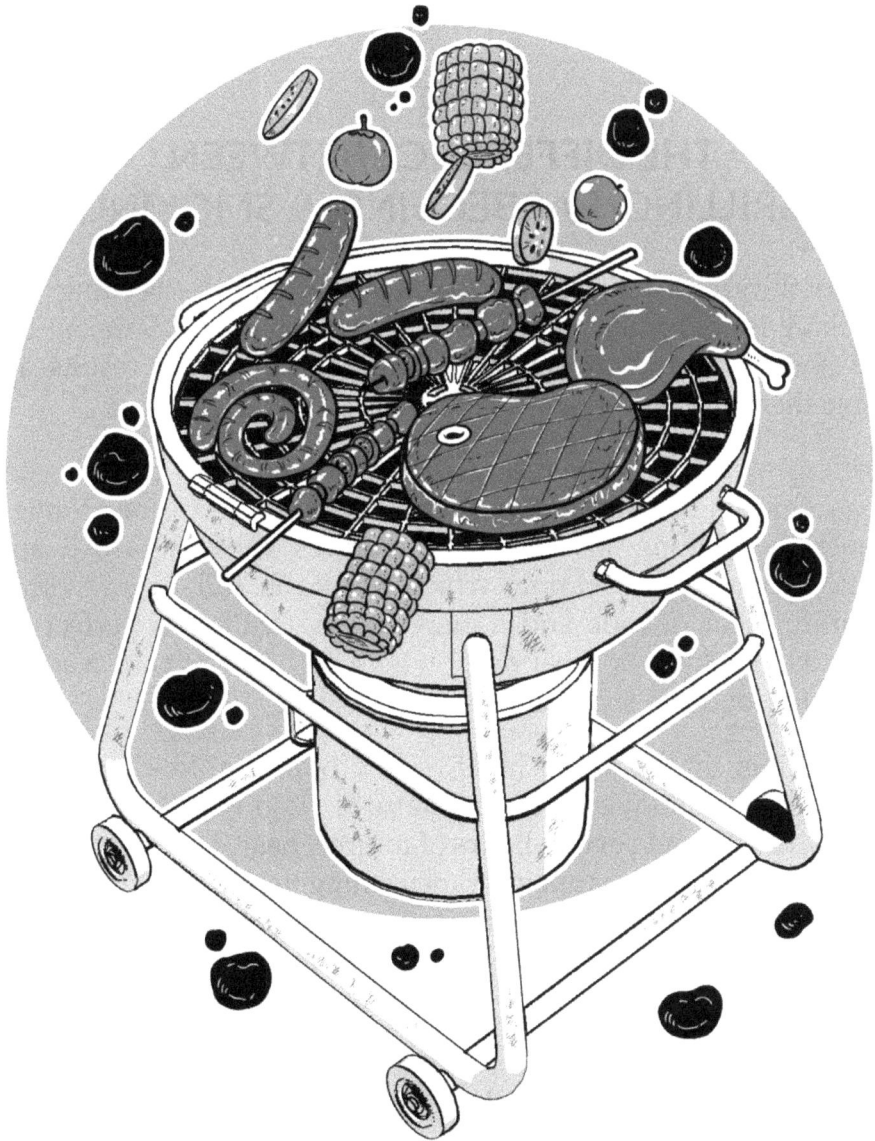

Every pitmaster, backyard warrior, and weekend griller has to start somewhere. Just as you can't build a castle without a good foundation, you can't become a BBQ legend without a firm grasp of the fundamentals. This chapter speaks to beginners who are just firing up their first grill and accomplished cooks who want to freshen up on the basics. The goal is to arm you with the confidence to know what you're doing before you even light the first match!

[1]
THE DIFFERENCE BETWEEN GRILLING, BARBECUING, & SMOKING

One of the greatest misconceptions is that grilling, barbecuing, and smoking is the same thing. This is far from the case. Sure, all use fire and meat, but the methods, temperatures, and results are altogether different.

Grilling means high heat and fast cooking. Think burgers, hot dogs, chicken breasts, and vegetables cooking over direct flames. Generally, grilling involves temperatures between 400°F and 600°F. There's also searing, which results in full flavor with a beautiful char outside and a juicy inside. Grilling is perfect for everyday cooking or meal prep, where no one wants to wait for hours for food at a social gathering.

Barbecuing, on the other hand, is the opposite: low and slow. Traditional techniques use temperatures ranging anywhere from 225°F to 275°F and several hours of indirect heat. This is where the magic of tenderness happens, transforming tough cuts like brisket, pork shoulder, and ribs into melt-in-your-mouth creations. Barbecuing is truly all about patience and pride. It's more about the journey than the destination.

Smoking is a technique for infusing meat with flavor from smoldering wood. Cold smoking (below 90°F) is used to flavor cheese, nuts, and fish. Meanwhile, hot smoking uses "regular"

BBQ temperatures. Smoking requires keeping a close eye on airflow, wood selection, and temperature stability.

In other words, grilling is speed, barbecuing is patience, and smoking is creativity. If you can get just these definitions right, you're already ahead of most home cooks.

[2]
CHOOSING THE RIGHT GRILL FOR YOU

The grill that's right for you depends on your grilling style, patience, and personality. Let's look at the three most common grill types.

CHARCOAL GRILLS

This classic, original grill is perfect for anyone looking to experience that primal feeling of being in charge of fire. Charcoal grills provide unbeatable smoky flavor and full control over heat zones. Charcoal grills are versatile, making them perfect for everything from high-heat burgers to low-and-slow BBQ.

Of course, the downside is that they require time and effort. This type of grill involves lighting charcoal, monitoring and transforming airflow, and maintaining stable temperatures. If you're the type of guy who appreciates the process as much as the end product, you'll take pride in a charcoal grill.

GAS GRILLS

When you want convenience, gas grills are the weekday BBQ warrior. Simply push a button to fire it up, and a few minutes later, you can be cooking. Quick and easy, they're great for casual dinners—or any time you don't feel like messing with lighting coals for twenty minutes.

However, cooking with gas means sacrificing the deep, smoky flavor you get with charcoal. As far as practicality goes, though, if you want a consistent winner with no fuss, gas is the way to go.

PELLET GRILLS

The new wave of BBQ technology, these grills use compressed wood pellets to burn charcoal, giving you that smoky fire flavor and the convenience of gas. Many come with digital controls, allowing you to choose a temperature setting and walk away as it holds steady heat.

The downside? Cost. Pellet grills can be expensive, and you'll need a good supply of pellets on hand. If you're interested in precision cooking with the flavor and atmosphere of smoke—and don't mind spending money—a pellet grill is absolutely the best choice.

Which of these grills sounds the most enticing?

Love tradition and ritual? Charcoal is for you.

Value convenience and speed? Gas is your friend.

Want flavor, control, and tech? Pellet is king.

[3]
ESSENTIAL FUEL CHOICES

Every good pitmaster knows his fuels. The fire you build determines flavor, consistency, and overall ability to execute your BBQ. Let's take a look at your choices: lump charcoal, briquettes, wood chips and chunks, and propane.

LUMP CHARCOAL

Lump charcoal is the purist's option. Made from chunks of actual hardwood, this fuel burns hot and clean, with less ash than briquettes. It imparts an unmistakable smokiness and allows you to control temperature with airflow. The downside to lump charcoal is that it burns faster than briquettes, so long cooks require refueling. However, if you're looking for flavor and authenticity, it's lump charcoal all the way.

BRIQUETTES

Briquettes are the workhorse of backyard BBQs. Briquettes are uniform, made from compacted charcoal dust, and often mixed with binders. They burn longer and more steadily than lumps, so briquettes are more reliable for slow and steady combustion. They're also wallet-friendly and easy to find. Purists may say that briquettes produce more ash and less flavor than lump, but many backyard pitmasters rely on their consistency.

WOOD CHIPS & CHUNKS

When it comes to smoking, wood is your main weapon. There are a variety of woods, each imparting a distinct combination of flavors:

- **Hickory:** Bold and bacon-y
- **Mesquite:** Strong and earthy
- **Apple:** Mild and sweet
- **Cherry:** Fruity and rich

Chips are advantageous for short cooks, while larger chunks and splits are best for long smokes. Don't be afraid to experiment with different combinations of wood until you find your own signature flavor!

PROPANE

If you're using a gas grill or smoker, propane will be your constant companion. Propane is a clean, readily available, and reliable source of heat. Of course, you won't get that smoky, natural flavor without a smoker box, but for convenience and control, propane is the way to go.

[4]
LIGHTING A GRILL WITHOUT BLOWING YOURSELF UP

Fire is both your BFF and your biggest enemy. Don't make the rookie mistake of pouring lighter fluid on charcoal until it looks like a bonfire. Sure, it's quick, but it'll ruin your meat and flavor it with nasty chemicals. That's not BBQ—it's sabotage, plain and simple. Each grill calls for a different strategy, so let's talk about how to light 'em up right!

FOR CHARCOAL GRILLS

A chimney starter is a metal cylinder that allows you to load your charcoal over a fire starter. In as little as fifteen minutes, you'll have glowing coals without using a single drop of lighter fluid.

Fire loves oxygen, so it's important to arrange your coals carefully. When lighting directly, stacking your coals in a pyramid shape will allow air to circulate. Don't take shortcuts. Using matches, lighters, or natural fire starters is fine, but avoid chemicals to preserve the taste of your meat.

FOR GAS GRILLS

Gas grills are easier and take less time, but don't underestimate them. Always open the lid before turning on the gas to prevent propane buildup. Otherwise, igniting your grill may result in a fireball. Once open, hit the ignition button or use a long lighter, and you're off to the races.

FOR PELLET GRILLS

Pellet grills are the easiest to light. Load the hopper, turn it on, and let the auger and igniter do the work. Don't get lazy, though. Keep the hopper clean, and make sure your pellets stay dry. There's nothing worse than soggy pellets, which clog the system and ruin your BBQ experience.

[5]
UNDERSTANDING
HEAT ZONES

Every man who wants to avoid burning the outside of a steak while leaving it raw inside needs to know the value of heat zones. Learning how to set up and implement heat zones will improve your cooking instantly.

DIRECT HEAT

Direct heat involves cooking over flame or hot coals to create the perfect sear. Burgers, steaks, kebabs, and hot dogs thrive here. Temperatures can exceed 500°F to 600°F. The downside is that leaving food on too long results in a charred, obliterated mess. Direct heat is about constant maintenance, so stay close, flip your food with confidence, and—above all—never leave your grill unattended.

INDIRECT HEAT

Using indirect heat means placing your food next to the flame instead of directly over it. Here, you can think of your grill like an oven. Temperatures usually range from 225°F to 350°F, perfect for large cuts like brisket, pork shoulders, and whole chickens. Indirect heat breaks connective tissue down without burning the outside, resulting in tender, evenly cooked meat.

TWO-ZONE SETUP

Here is the pitmaster's secret weapon: a two-zone fire. With charcoal, place a large pile of burning coals on one side of the grill, leaving the other side empty. With gas, turn the burners on one side of the grill while leaving the other side off. This setup provides versatility. You can sear your steak over direct heat, then transfer it to the cooler side for a gentle finish that eliminates problems with raw centers.

[6]
BASIC BBQ ETIQUETTE
FOR HOSTING

BBQ is about food, but it's also about people. When you supervise the grill, you're both the cook and the host. Of course, BBQ has its own rules, and if you observe them, you'll be a pitmaster people remember with fondness.

RULE 1: OWN THE GRILL

A grill is hallowed ground. Don't let every Joe with a beer in hand start jabbing your meat! Too many cooks will spoil more than the broth—they'll ruin your brisket. Receive advice graciously, but stay in control.

RULE 2: CONTROL THE DRINK

BBQ and beer go hand in hand, so you should make sure everyone, including yourself, has enough to drink. After all, hydration is important, especially as you stand over the heat of the grill. Keep a cooler nearby to avoid abandoning your post unnecessarily.

RULE 3: TIME IT RIGHT

Don't keep your guests waiting too long. While brisket can take twelve hours, a burger shouldn't take forty-five minutes. Providing snacks, sides, and appetizers helps entertain guests while the main event cooks, so plan ahead. After all, hungry guests are grumpy guests!

RULE 4: SERVE IT IN STYLE

When the food is ready, serve it with pride. Don't mumble, "I think this chicken is done." Instead, yell, "Wings are up! Dive in!" Confidence puts everyone at the table in a good mood.

RULE 5: CLEAN AS YOU GO

No one wants to see last week's grease stuck to your grates. A clean grill is a happy grill, and it also shows respect for your guests and your craft. BBQing is more than just flipping meat; you're creating an experience.

[7]
PATIENCE
IS KEY

If there's one difference between a real BBQ experience and a budget backyard meal, it's this: BBQ isn't fast food. You can't simply throw a sack of ribs on the grill and expect perfection in thirty minutes. Don't treat BBQ as a cheap alternative. View it as an entirely unique practice that requires time and patience. Luckily, when you love your grill, hours often feel like mere minutes, making BBQ more than worth the time investment.

For example, brisket is full of connective tissue that will resemble shoe leather if you treat it like steak. However, that same cut transforms into buttery, smoky goodness with half a day of slow, low heat. It's a miracle made possible with patience.

When you're barbecuing, you need to be conscious of the clock, the fire, the smoke, and watching the meat transition to a different texture. Every pitmaster knows about the "stall" — the absolute worst moment when your pork shoulder rises to a not-so-hot 160°F, then just hangs there. When this happens, newbie pitmasters often freak out and crank up the heat, ruining the meat. Veteran pitmasters, however, crack a cold one, wrap the meat in foil if necessary, and let time do its work.

Here's the reality: If you need a quick meal, BBQ isn't the hobby for you. If you want fall-off-the-bone ribs, pulled pork that falls apart, or brisket that makes grown men cry, you must commit. Like a good investment that pays dividends on discipline, BBQing pays a dividend on patience. You'll see the reward—as long as you're not in a hurry.

[8]
COMMON MYTHS
DEBUNKED

The world of BBQ is plagued by bad advice and persistent myths swapped at the water cooler or passed from bar to bar. Let's debunk a of these right here and now.

MYTH 1: FLIP YOUR MEAT ONLY ONCE

Some backyard "experts" will tell you that one flip is sufficient—and if you do more, you'll ruin your steak or burger. That is simply not true; multiple flips can actually create more uniform cooking. What's important isn't the number of flips but how often you flip and the temperature of your fire.

MYTH 2: PRESSING DOWN ON BURGERS MAKES THEM JUICIER

When you squish a burger with a spatula, you're essentially squeezing all the juices out and onto the coals. Congratulations, you just exchanged flavor for a puff of smoke! The juiciest burgers result from a gentle touch, so don't smash.

MYTH 3: PINK EQUALS RAW

Color isn't necessarily an indication of doneness. Smoked meats often have a pink "smoke ring" around the edges, which is evidence that you did it right. The only way to determine whether meat is safe to eat is to use a thermometer. Chicken should reach 165°F, pork requires a minimum of 145°F, and beef varies based on preference.

MYTH 4: MORE SMOKE EQUALS MORE FLAVOR

Too much smoke will make your food taste like an ashtray. The goal is to create thin blue smoke, not huge white clouds. If it looks like a tire fire, you're doing it wrong. To achieve mouthwatering results that carry the table, you must learn the science behind BBQ and respect the process.

[9]
BUILDING YOUR
BBQ PLAYLIST

While you're cooking, a good playlist is vital to set the right tone. Choose music that can ride the rhythm of the smoke, keeping you company and setting the mood for your guests. So what makes a perfect BBQ soundtrack?

CLASSIC ROCK

Nothing screams backyard BBQ louder than Lynyrd Skynyrd, AC/DC, or ZZ Top. You can't go wrong with guitar riffs while you're smoking ribs.

BLUES

Slow and soulful blues can complement the low-and-slow cooking tempo. Try incorporating B.B. King or Muddy Waters into your soundtrack when cooking brisket.

COUNTRY

Historically, BBQ and country music are thick as thieves. Songs about whiskey, trucks, and good times provide a perfect backdrop for cooking pulled pork.

REGGAE

To set a summer BBQ vibe, nothing pairs with a cold beer like the laid-back beats of Bob Marley or Peter Tosh.

HIP-HOP OR R&B

If you prefer something more modern, smooth hip-hop or R&B tunes will keep things upbeat while maintaining the chill factor.

The magic is in the balance. At the beginning of your day, when you're tending the smoker, pick something easy and steady. Then, when the party kicks in and there's food ready to go, turn up the energy. Music is part of the memory your guests will hold long after the last bone is licked clean.

[10]
THE ROLE OF BEER
IN BBQ

Now, let's dive into the liquid that fuels every good cookout: beer.

HYDRATION

Standing over a hot grill can be a sweaty affair. Beer helps keep you cool, refreshed, and patient during long waits. It's a tradition. However, like anything else, moderation is key. You're the one in charge of a fire, after all. Drink responsibly.

BEER PAIRING WITH BBQ

Choosing the right beer involves pairing flavors, and different beers work better with certain meats:

> **Light lagers or pilsners:** Light, crisp, and refreshing brews are perfectly suited to chicken or seafood.

> **IPAs:** Bold and hoppy, IPAs go well with spicy ribs or smoked sausage.

Stouts and porters: Rich and malty, stouts and porters stand up nicely to brisket or pulled pork.

Wheat beers: Smooth and subtly sweet, wheat varieties are ideal companions to vegetables or lighter BBQ fare.

COOKING WITH BEER

Beer can also be used in marinades or sauces and provides a steaming liquid for sausages. For example, to make beer-can chicken, shove an open beer into a whole bird and stick it on the grill. The steam keeps the chicken moist while the skin crisps.

CHAPTER TWO: TOOLS OF THE TRADE

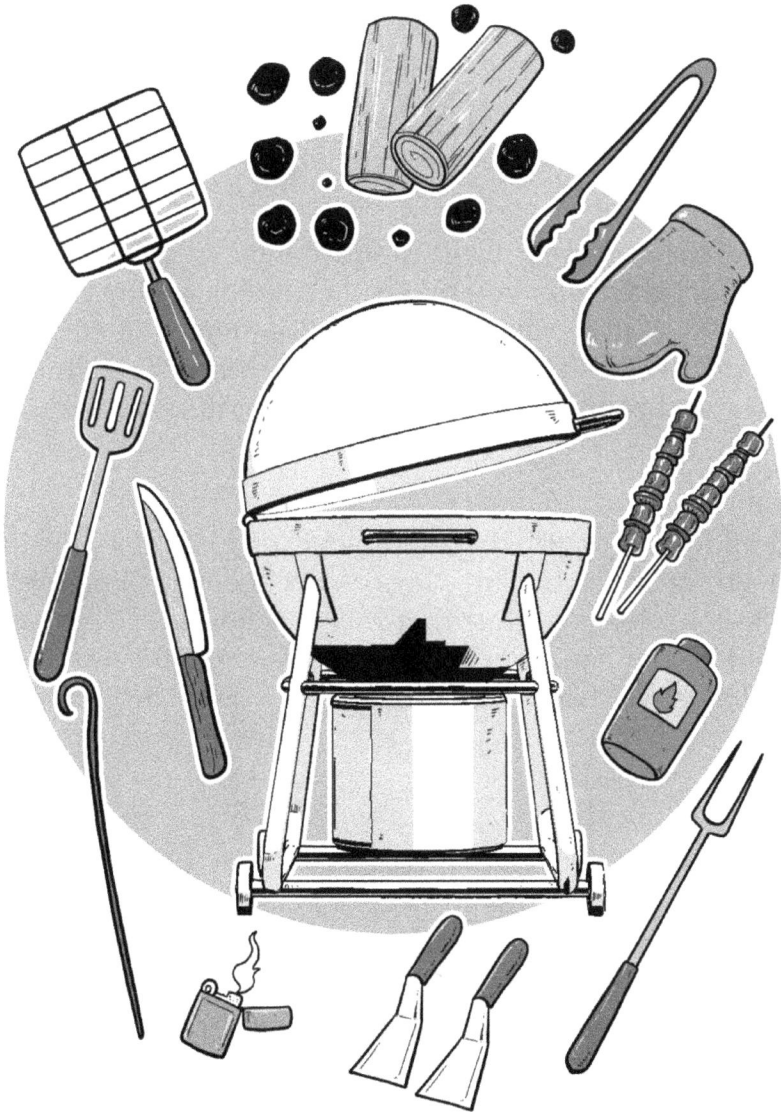

A pitmaster is only as good as his equipment. You can have the best cuts of meat on Earth and the hottest fire in town, but it won't matter if you're flipping steaks with a butter knife and applying sauce with a paintbrush you found in the garage. You don't have to break the bank to get the right tools. With a few solid investments, you can build a BBQ arsenal that covers everything from burgers to brisket.

[11]
MUST HAVE
TOOLS

Don't go chasing fancy devices and gimmicks as you shop for tools. In fact, there are only four essential tools a pitmaster needs to preside over the coals. These four tools—tongs, spatula, brush, and thermometer—are absolute requirements. Take their use seriously, and your guests will thank you for it.

TONGS

Tongs allow you to grip, flip, and move food without puncturing it and letting important drippings escape. Look for long-handled stainless-steel tongs with spring-lock functionality. They should feel solid in your hand, not like flimsy versions in the discount bin. Cheap tongs will bend, break, or—even worse—drop your food directly into the flames.

SPATULA

Not just for burgers, a proper spatula with a large, flat surface is necessary for flipping fish, lifting a delicate veggie, or rescuing a chicken wing that's dangerously close to the edge of the grill. A spatula with a beveled edge is easier to slide underneath items, and a longer handle will save your knuckles from scorching.

BRUSH

BBQ creates a mess, and that's part of the fun. Of course, this means you need a good basting brush to spread your sauces adequately while keeping your grates clean. Look for a basting brush with silicone bristles, as silicone is easy to wash and more durable than old-fashioned bristles.

THERMOMETER

Real men use thermometers. Period. No one can tell if meat is done by poking it with their finger like some steak oracle. That's how you end up with chicken that's raw in the center or pork that's dried up. Your best option is a digital instant-read thermometer; nothing has changed the barbecue game more than this handy gadget.

[12]
INVESTING IN A
GOOD GRILL BRUSH

Here's an absolute fact: A nasty grill is a downright disservice to BBQ. Stale, charred remnants do not add "flavor." They'll ruin your meal instead. Since a clean grill is essential, you need the right brush to do the job properly.

Wire-bristle grill brushes have been the preferred tool for years, and they do scour caked-on grime with ease. But those tiny pieces of wire often break off, sticking to the grates and ending up in your food. No one will appreciate biting into a burger with a wayward wire in it. When that happens, not only is dinner ruined, but you might be making an unplanned visit to the ER too.

Here's what you should be using instead:

> **Bristle-less grill brushes:** Coils of stainless steel or scrapers can achieve the same result without leaving wire bristles on your grill.

Grill scrapers: Most scrapers are made of wood or stainless steel. They're either entirely flat or shaped to match the grooves of the grill grates.

Grill stones or pads: These basic cleaning tools are made from pumice or similar materials. They wear down as they clean, but leave nothing dangerous behind.

PRO TIP: CLEAN IT WHILE IT'S HOT

As a best practice, the ideal time to clean your grill is while the grates are still hot. Heat helps loosen the grease, making it easier to scrape off. Think of it like brushing your teeth: You wouldn't wait a week to clean your teeth, so don't leave junk to collect until you cook again.

Investing in a safe and effective grill brush isn't being picky; it's protecting your guests, your food, and your reputation. After all, no one will remember how perfectly you grilled their steak if it's served with a side of wire.

[13]
CHIMNEY STARTERS VS. LIGHTER FLUID

Let's settle one of the oldest arguments in backyard BBQ: the best way to light your coals. If you're still soaking briquettes in lighter fluid, it's time for a wake-up call.

THE CASE AGAINST LIGHTER FLUID

Sure, lighter fluid is an easy way to light your coals, but there's a big downside: flavor. Those chemicals don't just burn away. They settle into your food, and nothing derails your rib game faster than a mouthful of chemicals.

THE ADVANTAGE OF A CHIMNEY STARTER

A chimney starter is the way forward in the BBQ world. It's basically a simple metal cylinder with a grate at the bottom. You fill the chimney with charcoal, stuff a starter in the bottom, and light it. Airflow does its thing, and in fifteen minutes, you have a tower of red-hot coals to pour into your grill without any chemicals or unusual flavors.

PRO TIPS FOR USING A CHIMNEY STARTER

Use natural fire starters: Crumpled newspaper works, but wax cubes and paraffin starters burn longer and make this process foolproof.

Don't overfill: Remember that fire needs oxygen to thrive. If you pack your chimney too full, the coals will take forever to ignite. Two-thirds full is generally a safe bet.

Pour carefully: When the coals are ready, handle them appropriately. Use heat-resistant gloves and pour at a steady pace into your grill.

Once you switch to chimney starters, you'll never go back. This cleaner, safer option to starting your fire will make it obvious that you know your stuff.

[14]
SMOKERS—OFFSET, VERTICAL, OR ELECTRIC?

Every BBQ king will eventually have a moment of reckoning: Is it time to get a smoker? Grills are versatile beasts, but smokers always rank best for cooking low and slow. That leg of lamb, tender brisket, or fall-apart pork shoulder requires hours of controlled smoke. That being said, smokers come in many varieties, so which is right for you?

OFFSET SMOKERS

These are the heavyweights of the BBQ world. Think of a horizontal barrel with a firebox attached to the side. With an offset smoker, heat and smoke drift from the firebox into the main chamber, indirectly cooking your meat. The pros are authentic smoke flavor and plenty of room for large cuts. Plus, just owning one will make you look like you know what you're doing.

However, using an offset smoker is also a hands-on activity. You'll be babysitting your fire, constantly adjusting airflow, and adding wood every hour. If you like the ritual of tending to a fire with a beer nearby, great! If not, it'll just be exhausting.

VERTICAL SMOKERS

Often referred to as "bullet smokers," vertical smokers are essentially a tower with a fire chamber at the bottom, a water pan at the middle, and cooking racks above. The pan helps regulate temperature and prevent the meat from drying out.

Bullet smokers are affordable and surprisingly efficient. They're perfect for beginners who want real smoke flavor without the price tag of an offset. The downside is that they have a limited surface area for cooking. Don't expect to smoke a whole hog with this type of smoker.

ELECTRIC SMOKERS

An electric smoker is the easiest option. Simply plug it in, add wood chips, set the temperature, and walk away. The smoker does the rest. They're great for beginners or anyone short on time.

On the other hand, purists will scoff. Electric smokers don't produce an "authentic" smoke flavor and lack the romance of tending to a fire. It's all about your priorities. If you just want to set it and forget it, electric is the way to go.

[15]
ACCESSORIES

Once you've got the basic necessities, consider adding some accessories to take your BBQ to the next level. Far from gimmicks, practical add-ons can make life easier and allow experimentation with new techniques.

GRILL MATS

Ever grilled shrimp or asparagus and watched them drop through the grates? That's where grill mats come into play. These heat-resistant mats go over your grates, providing a flat cooking surface while allowing smoke and heat through. They're best for small or delicate foods like veggies, fish, or even eggs. Pro tip? Don't use with super intense flames; mats work best at medium heat.

GRILL BASKETS

Think of grill baskets as cages for your food. These metal baskets can hold anything from veggies to chicken wings to diced potatoes. Using them is simple: Toss your food in and close the basket. You can flip the whole basket at once—no more chasing peppers around the grill with your tongs. Decent grill baskets are available for as little as $20, and they last for years.

ROTISSERIE

This is the king of accessories. Attach a rotisserie kit to your BBQ and load it with a whole chicken, leg, or lamb, or a prime rib. Then let that baby rotate over open fire. Rotation continually bastes the meat in its natural juices, resulting in perfect tenderness and crispy skin.

The key is to always balance the load.

[16]
KNIFE SKILLS
FOR BBQ

A pitmaster without a good knife is like a sniper without a scope. Hacking and tearing meat with a dull or inappropriate blade is an amateur move. With the proper tool, though, you can look like a pro while providing the perfect slice.

ESSENTIAL BBQ KNIVES

Chef's knife (8 to 10 inches): Your go-to for just about everything, from chopping onions to trimming fat off brisket.

Boning knife: Thin and flexible, ideal for trimming fat and silver skin or separating ribs.

Carving knife or slicer: Allows for nice, clean slices of brisket, turkey, or roast.

Cleaver (optional): Good for breaking down big cuts or hacking through a bone.

SHARPENING MATTERS

It may seem counterintuitive, but a dull knife can be more dangerous than a sharp one. A dull blade requires more force, increasing the likelihood of slipping. Invest in a sharpening steel or whetstone, and learn proper technique to keep your knives honed.

SAFETY & TECHNIQUE

As you cook, follow these three core rules:

- Always cut on a stable surface. A wobbly cutting board is a

  recipe for disaster.

- Always use the right knife for the job. Don't try to carve brisket with a paring knife.

- Practice. Clean, even slices are more attractive and ensure equal portions.

A sharp, presentable knife set doesn't have to break the bank. You can build a good arsenal for about $100. Make your blades last by hand washing, storing properly, and sharpening regularly. Knives are tools, not toys, so respect your blades and they'll serve you faithfully for a long time.

[17]
APRONS, GLOVES & MANLY BBQ APPAREL

As you know, BBQ is a messy business. Any time you deal with smoke, grease, sauce, and fire, you're bound to get dirty. Before you sacrifice your favorite shirt to the BBQ gods, consider investing in protective gear that makes you look like a BBQ stud.

APRONS

Throw out those cutesy aprons in favor of quality and functionality. Quality aprons are made from heavy-duty canvas or leather. A good apron protects your clothes from grease splatters, flare-ups, and drippy sauces. It should also have various pockets for meat thermometers, tongs, or even a cold beer. Lastly, a rugged-looking apron doesn't need a silly saying to communicate what it is (unless that's your preference).

GLOVES

Naked skin is no match for a 500°F grill grate. Therefore, gloves are a must-have and a vast improvement over run-of-the-mill oven mitts. There are two types of gloves:

> **Heat-resistant gloves (either silicone or Kevlar):** Great for handling hot grates, pans, or hot coals

> **Disposable food-safe gloves (nitrile):** Ideal for keeping your hands grease-free while trimming meat, applying rubs, or pulling a pork shoulder apart

In cold environments, use nitrile gloves over cotton liner gloves to keep your hands warm without sacrificing dexterity.

MANLY BBQ CLOTHING

You don't need a special outfit to grill, but quality apparel keeps you safe and comfortable. Think breathable fabrics, closed-toe shoes, and a hat to block the sun. You get extra credit for a shirt that you're not worried about staining. After all, it adds character. At the end of the day, BBQ garb is about both safety and style. Instead of "four-star chef," you're going more for "commander of fire."

[18]
DIGITAL VS. ANALOG THERMOMETERS

We've mentioned thermometers, but now, let's take a closer look. Precision is the difference between a juicy success and a nasty, dry mess. You may have heard the common saying, "Cook it until it feels done." This is a rookie move, though. A true pitmaster uses a thermometer. The real question is whether you should use a digital or an analog thermometer.

ANALOG THERMOMETERS

Analog thermometers are true dial thermometers. Shove it in, wait for the needle to move, and make your call. They're cheap, simple, and don't require batteries.

- **Pros:** Good, affordable, reliable in rugged situations
- **Cons:** Slow, less accurate, difficult to read in low light

DIGITAL THERMOMETERS

The contemporary tool of choice, digital instant-read thermometers, provide a temperature in seconds, usually to a tenth of a degree. Some even come with leave-in probes that allow you to monitor the meat wirelessly as it cooks via an app on your phone.

- **Pros:** Quick, accurate, intuitive, and fantastic for multitasking
- **Cons:** Pricey, requires batteries

[19]
STORAGE & ORGANIZATION FOR YOUR BBQ ARSENAL

True pitmasters would never dream of piling their tools in the corner, tossing them in a random drawer, or leaving them to rust on a cold grill. Your tools deserve respect, and organizing your pit or station makes life easier and saves you money since you won't be replacing lost or damaged tools as often.

Toolbox and totes: A simple toolbox is effective for keeping your tongs, spatula, brushes, and thermometers together and ready to go. You can even find BBQ-specific totes with slots for each unique tool.

Magnetic strips and hooks: Mounting a magnetic strip on the side of your grill or in your garage is a perfect way to keep track of metal tools, while hooks are ideal for hanging aprons, gloves, or baskets.

Storage bins for fuel: Never store charcoal or pellets in open bags. Moisture will ruin them. Airtight containers are vital to keep your fuel in top shape. Make sure to label each container so that you don't accidentally grab lump charcoal when you're looking for applewood chunks.

THE RITUAL OF READINESS

Every pitmaster has a ritual: sharpening knives, refilling bins, and restocking sauces. Organization isn't boring; it's part of the craft. When everything has its place, you can focus on planning your meal and prepping your grill.

[20]
DIY HACKS TO UPGRADE ON A BUDGET

Not all BBQ upgrades need a significant investment. With a little creativity, you can hack your equipment and setup to elevate your grilling and smoking experiences. The legacy of BBQ is by no means measured in monetary value; it resides in the love you put into your craft. With a bit of ingenuity and DIY spirit, you can make your BBQ gear work for you without spending your entire paycheck.

DIY FIRE PIT & SMOKER

Want a second grill? Stack fire-safe bricks in a square, rest a piece of grating across it, and you have a makeshift BBQ pit. It may look a bit funny, but this setup is ideal for camping or backyard science experiments. Don't have a smoker? No problem! Use a small metal box (or even tinfoil) with holes poked through it instead.

REPURPOSE, REUSE, RECYCLE

- **Meat injector:** Ever wondered why meat injectors have to be so expensive? Not to worry. A turkey baster with a needle attachment will do the job in a pinch.
- **Baking sheets:** Use your old baking sheets as a drip pan.
- **Old pans:** Break out your cast iron pans for grilling vegetables or even cornbread.
- **Tin cans:** Punch out some holes and fill the cans with wood chips for a disposable smoker box.

CHAPTER THREE:
MEAT MASTERY

If fire is the soul of BBQ, then meat is its beating heart. You can have the best utensils and the most patient disposition, but if you don't know your cuts, you'll always be climbing uphill. Meat selection isn't just grabbing whatever looks good at the grocery store. It involves knowing which cuts will shine on the grill, which need low-and-slow cooking for hours, and which require special attention to ensure they don't dry out. Let's break down the holy trinity of BBQ: beef, pork, and poultry.

[21]
BEST CUTS OF
BEEF FOR BBQ

Beef and BBQ are matched like smoke and fire. However, not all beef is created equal. The difference between legendary brisket and a chewy disaster is knowing how to select the proper cut.

BRISKET

Brisket is the king of BBQ. Brisket comes from the lower chest of the cow. It's a very active muscle with lots of connective tissue. It looks tough and unappetizing, but that's exactly what makes it perfect for BBQ. When cooked low and slow, collagen breaks down into gelatin, transforming tough meat into a flavorful, juicy work of art.

- **Cooking:** Smoke low and slow at 225°F to 250°F for ten to fourteen hours. An internal temperature of 203°F is perfect for a soft texture.
- **Cutting:** Always slice brisket against the grain. Otherwise, you'll ruin hours of hard work.

RIBS

Few cuts of beef shout "BBQ" louder than a rack of ribs. Crowds absolutely love these meaty, flavorful cuts, and they look amazing on the plate. There are two major types of ribs:

- **Back ribs:** Smaller, with less actual meat, back ribs are cut closer to the spine
- **Short ribs:** Thick and loaded with beefy flavor
- **Cooking:** Both grilling and low-and-slow smoking are great options. The 3-2-1 method (3 hours smoking, 2 hours wrapped, and 1 hour sauced) works every time.

STEAK

Not all steaks are ideal for grilling, but the best steaks take themselves to the grill. Ribeye, strip, T-bone, and porterhouse steaks all have great marbling and tenderness.

- **Cooking:** Fast sear over high heat and call it a day. Medium rare (130°F to 135°F) is best for locking in as much juice as possible.
- **Pro tip:** Let steaks rest for at least five minutes after grilling. Cut too soon and you'll pull the plug on all those delicious juices.

[22]
PORK PERFECTION

Pork is the workhorse of BBQ. It's adaptable, affordable, and usually doesn't require much experience. From pulled pork sandwiches to sticky ribs, pork provides comfort food at its tasty, smoky best.

PORK SHOULDER (BOSTON BUTT)

This cut comes from the upper shoulder. Generally tough and fatty, this meat is perfect for low-and-slow cooking. With time and patience, pork shoulder will transform into pulled pork that practically shreds itself.

- **Cooking:** Smoke at 225°F to 250°F for eight to twelve hours. The right temperature range for a perfect shred is around 195°F to 205°F.

- **Pro tip:** For faster cooking, wrap in foil or butcher paper at the stall around 160°F to retain moisture.

PORK LOIN

Pork loin is leaner, starting at the front of the loin and running down to the pig's back. It's tender and mild in flavor but easily dries out if cooked too long.

- **Cooking:** Pork loin is best grilled or roasted with indirect heat. Pull out at 145°F for juicy slices.
- **Pro tip:** Brine pork loin in a solution of salt and sugar before cooking to hold moisture and add flavor.

BABY BACK RIBS

Baby back ribs are cut from the top of the ribcage, close to the spine. Shorter and leaner than spare ribs, baby backs are loved for their tenderness.

- **Cooking:** Cook low and slow, often using the 3-2-1 method.
- **Pro tip:** Remove the membrane before cooking, as it can be tough and block the good smoke.

[23]
CHICKEN & TURKEY

Here's the deal: Despite what you may have heard, cooking poultry can be confusing. One mistake and you're left with a dry, boring disaster that no sauce can save. Fortunately, we're here to give you the down and dirty. Chicken and turkey might not possess the boldness of beef or the comfort of pork, but do it right, and poultry will gain a permanent place in your BBQ rotation.

CHICKEN

Chicken is a popular choice for BBQ because it's affordable and fast. However, chicken is tricky, particularly white meat (e.g., chicken breast), and will dry out quickly if you're not careful.

- **Cooking:** Grill thighs, legs, and wings over direct heat, watching for crispy skin. You can smoke or roast whole chickens at 275°F to 300°F.
- **Pro tip:** Spatchcock your chicken by cutting out the backbone and flattening the bird for even cooking, great moisture, and crispy skin.

TURKEY

Turkey isn't just for Thanksgiving — it's excellent for BBQ as well. Of course, it suffers from the same problem as chicken: dryness.

- **Cooking:** Smoke whole turkeys at 275°F. You might want to separate the breast and legs, though, for even and thorough cooking.
- **Pro tip:** Keep it simple by brining your bird. A basic saltwater brine (with herbs, citrus, or sugar, if desired) will retain moisture in your bird. Bonus points if you inject hot flavored butter underneath the skin before smoking!

GENERAL POULTRY COOKING TIPS

- Cook all poultry to an internal temperature of 165°F.
- Don't rely on sauce to save a dry bird! Moisture starts with technique.
- Allow meat to rest before carving so that juices have time to redistribute.

[24]
SEAFOOD ON
THE GRILL

When most people think of BBQ, the first things that come to mind are ribs, brisket, or chicken wings. Seafood, however, provides an opportunity to display a different skill set and wow your guests. Seafood is quick, flavorful, and adds a beachy feel to summer cookouts. The trick is keeping it from sticking, falling apart, or drying out.

FISH

While fish fillets and steaks are fragile and will break apart if you mishandle them, they may surprise you when grilled properly. Salmon, tuna, swordfish, halibut, and snapper are all firm and can withstand grilling. Avoid thin, flaky fish like tilapia unless you're using a basket or foil.

- **Cooking:** Coat both the fish and grates in oil, then grill fillets on medium heat for three to four minutes per side until they flake with a fork.
- **Pro tip:** Leave the skin on to act as a natural barrier against heat and provide flavor.

SHRIMP

In addition to being super easy and quick, grilling shrimp is a surefire way to please the crowd. They're also a great vehicle for marinades.

- **Cooking:** Skewer shrimp or use a grill basket so that they don't fall through the grates. Cook shrimp on medium-high heat for two to three minutes per side. Watch carefully as it curls; you're looking for a C, so if you end up with an O-shaped shrimp, you've overcooked it.
- **Pro tip:** Add a garlic-butter baste while grilling to make your shrimp unforgettable.

OTHER SEAFOOD

Seafood may not be the first thing that comes to mind when you throw something on the grill, but it adds variety, elegance, and a lighter option for guests who aren't looking to eat heavy.

- **Scallops:** Scallops are sweet, tender, and only need about two minutes per side on a hot grill.
- **Lobster:** Split tails lengthwise, brush with butter, and grill shell-side down until the meat is opaque.
- **Clams and mussels:** Toss on the grill until they pop open for a salty, smoky punch that makes a great appetizer.

[25]
GAME MEATS FOR
THE ADVENTUROUS

For the pitmaster prepared to step beyond the butcher block, game meats are the ultimate challenge: daring, lean, and flavorful. However, game meats require skill—screw up, and you'll be left with nothing but chewy, dry disappointment.

VENISON

Deer meat is lean, which means it cooks quickly. As a result, venison dries out quickly when overcooked. Look for backstrap (the tenderloin of venison) and steaks. Ground venison also makes great burgers.

- **Cooking:** Use a marinade for moisture, then grill hot and fast to medium rare. Venison really does not like to be overcooked.
- **Pro tip:** Wrap venison steaks with bacon to add fat and flavor. This will also reduce the risk of dryness.

WILD BOAR

Wild boar is richer and darker than traditional pork, with a nutty, earthy flavor. Use shoulders for slow cooking and loins for quick grilling.

- **Cooking:** Treat wild boar as a hybrid between pork and beef. For loins, grill hot and fast; make sure to smoke shoulders long and low until the connective tissue breaks down.
- **Pro tip:** Wild boar is lean, so brining or marinating will always be good. A red wine base is effective for bringing out the depth of flavor.

OTHER OPTIONS

- **Duck:** Duck is fatty and flavorful. It's best grilled breast-down to render the fat.
- **Rabbit:** Rabbit is lean and subtle. It's best marinated, then grilled softly with indirect heat.

[26]
TRIM FAT & SILVER SKIN
LIKE A PRO

You can buy the best cuts of meat, but if you don't set them properly, you'll never get favorable results. Removing fat and silver skin is a behind-the-scenes skill that separates hobbyists from real pitmasters.

FAT TRIMMING

Not all fat is bad. In fact, fat equals flavor, but too much—or the wrong kind—will ruin the cook.

- **Beef Brisket:** Trim the fat cap down to about a quarter of an inch. Too thick, and the fat won't render; too thin, and the meat will be dry.

- **Pork Shoulder:** Cut away large, hard lumps of fat that won't render during cooking, leaving enough marbling to retain moisture.
- **Pro tip:** Use a sharp boning knife and trim it cold, when it's firm and easy to manage.

SILVER SKIN

Silver skin is that thin, silvery membrane found on ribs, tenderloin, and pork loin. Unlike fat, silver skin won't render. It just gets chewy and nasty. To remove it, slide the tip of a sharp knife under one edge, then grip the membrane with a single-use paper towel and pull away in one motion. With practice, you'll come away with one satisfying, continuous piece.

WHY IT MATTERS

Trimming meat isn't just about presentation. Properly trimmed meat cooks consistently, accepts rubs and marinades better, and provides the tender mouthful you're seeking. Trimming is one of those things nobody recognizes when you get it right, but they'll certainly notice when you do a poor job!

[27]
BRINING BASICS FOR JUICY RESULTS

One of the biggest offenses in BBQ circles is dry meat. Enter the pitmaster's secret weapon: brining. In its simplest terms, brining is soaking meat in a solution of saltwater. It's science at its finest. Salt transforms muscle fibers in meat, allowing them to hold more water. Translation: moist meat, even if you inadvertently overcook it slightly.

The basic formula for a brine is one gallon of water, one cup of kosher salt, and half a cup of sugar. Optional ingredients include garlic, fresh herbs, and citrus. The best meats for brining include poultry (especially turkey), pork chops, loins, and seafood like shrimp. Beef doesn't really need brining due to its natural fat content.

Small cuts, such as pork chops, take two to four hours. Whole chickens need eight to twelve hours. Turkey? A full twenty-four hours. Make sure to wash your meat and pat it dry after pulling it from the brine. Nobody wants a salt bomb!

[28]
AGING MEAT
AT HOME

Aging isn't just for wine and whiskey. Properly aging meat develops a stronger flavor and better tenderness. There are two primary forms: wet and dry aging.

WET AGING

Most supermarket meat is wet-aged. Basically, cuts of meat are vacuum-packed in plastic and rested for a couple of weeks. The meat's natural enzymes break down muscle fibers and improve tenderness. It's convenient, economical, and adds a light flavor.

- **Pros:** Easy to do, inexpensive, and readily available
- **Cons:** Doesn't pack the flavor punch of dry-aged meat

DRY AGING

Dry-aged meat is the holy grail. First, meat is kept exposed to air in a controlled environment with cool temperature, consistent humidity, and good airflow for two to six weeks. As the meat rests, the exterior dries and forms a crust. Then this outer crust is removed, leaving behind concentrated flavor that produces rich, buttery beef.

- **Pros:** Rich, nutty, and complex flavor

- **Cons:** Requires special equipment (or at least a dedicated fridge with airflow) and patience

At home, wet aging is the easier option. All you need is vacuum-sealed meat and patience. Dry aging takes commitment, but if you're serious about it, a small dry-aging fridge will take your steak from good to incredible.

[29]
SOURCING
QUALITY MEAT

Where you buy your meat matters. You may as well forget about cooking awesome BBQ without the right cuts.

SUPERMARKETS

While convenient and generally cheap, supermarket selections are limited. Cuts are pre-prepared and wrapped in plastic. Even worse, they may have been frozen and thawed in cold storage for weeks. Supermarkets are perfectly acceptable for a weeknight grill, but if you're cooking for a crowd, you'll want more options and control.

LOCAL BUTCHERS

Butchers are a pitmaster's best friends. Not only do they know their cuts, but they also source meat from local farms. Want a proper brisket with a nice, fat cap or a custom sausage blend? Butchers will prep the cuts as you request, and they can even share useful tips about meat prep. All you need to do is ask, and you'll learn tricks a supermarket guy probably wouldn't know.

For casual cooks, supermarkets are fine. If you're serious about grilling, however, one of the best things you can do is develop a relationship with a local butcher. They'll make sure you're making the best choices when you buy.

[30]
VEGETARIAN OPTIONS THAT WON'T EMBARRASS YOU

Somebody at your BBQ is going to be a vegetarian or at least trying to cut back on their meat consumption. While BBQ is basically all about fire and protein, a good host provides options. Don't fret. You can keep it vegetarian without losing your man card. After all, nothing brings veggies to life like the grill!

GRILLED VEGETABLES

- **Corn on the cob:** Slather with butter, sprinkle lightly with spices, and char until smoky goodness is achieved.
- **Peppers, zucchini, and eggplant:** Slice thick, brush with olive oil, and grill until softened.
- **Mushrooms:** Portobellos are particularly suited for the grill. They're meaty, smoky, and can even serve as a stand-in for burgers.

PLANT-BASED MEATS

The canonical list of plant-based items has expanded dramatically in the past few years. Now, for example, bean, soy, and pea-based burgers can be grilled just like a beef patty: season, sear, and make sure not to overcook.

Serve vegetarian dishes with confidence. Don't treat them like an afterthought or "lesser" dish. Sometimes, grilled vegetables or plant-based mains can even be better than a meat-focused one.

CHAPTER FOUR: FLAVORS THAT WIN

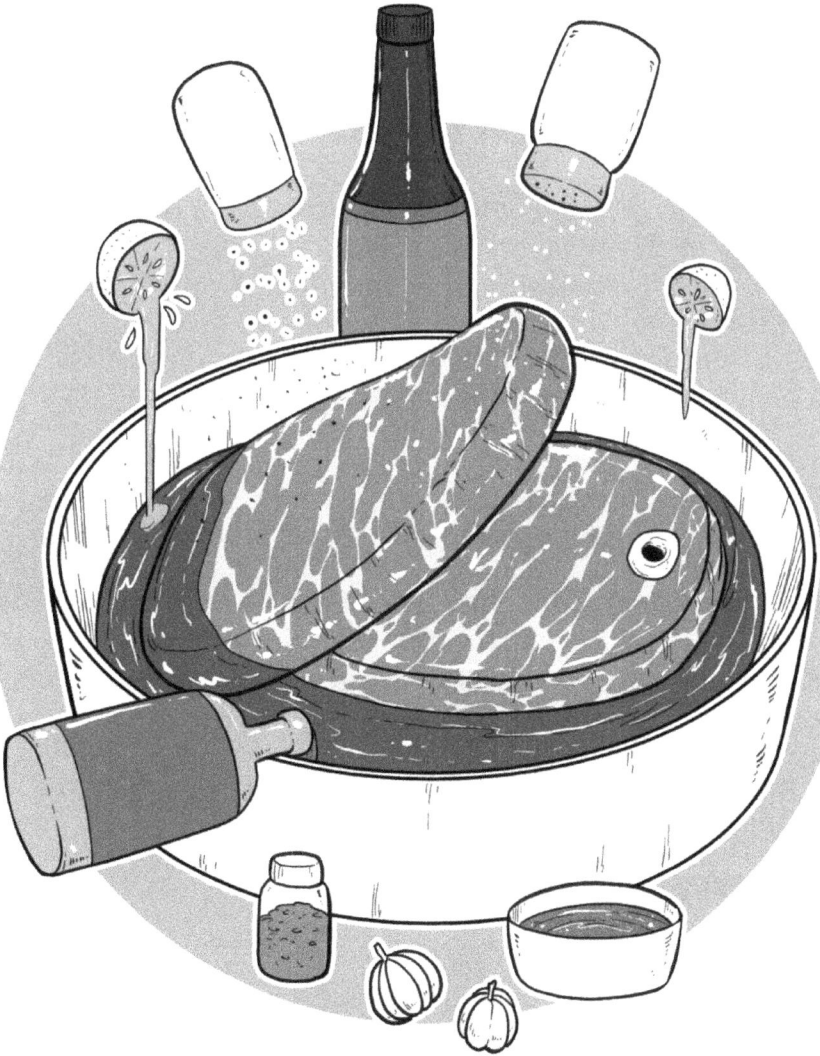

Meat plays a starring role in BBQ, but flavor is what brings people back for more. You might bring a brisket to the smoke house for fourteen hours, but if the seasoning is one-dimensional, your lines for seconds will be nonexistent. Great BBQ is about layering flavor—rubs, marinades, and sauces combined with smoke and the meat itself.

[31]
SWEET, SPICY, OR SAVORY DRY RUBS

If smoke is the best friend of BBQ, then dry rub is a handshake, the initial layer of flavor before meat hits the grill. A rub is about forming a crust, or *bark*, that locks juice in and provides an extra punch in each bite.

THE ELEMENTS OF A DRY RUB

Salt: Salt is the base. It elevates natural flavors while drawing moisture to the surface to form a crust. Kosher salt is best because it sticks well and retains good surface area.

Sugar: Sugar adds sweetness for caramelization. Brown sugar is a BBQ fan favorite, but beware. If you use too much, it might burn, especially over direct flame.

Spices: Paprika, garlic powder, onion powder, cumin, chili powder, cayenne—the list goes on and on. Spices provide complexity, heat, and depth to your meat.

THREE TYPES OF DRY RUBS

Sweet rubs: Basic sweet rubs use a brown sugar base combined with a dash of mild chili powder and paprika. They're ideal for pork ribs and chicken, where caramelized crust performs at its best.

Spicy rubs: Spicy rubs include cayenne, black pepper, chili flakes, and mustard powder. They're best on beef or other large, bold cuts that can take the heat.

Savory rubs: Savory rubs are comprised of garlic, onion, herbs, and smoked paprika to create a balanced type of earthy flavor. They're perfect for brisket or turkey.

PRO TIPS

Apply dry rubs at least thirty minutes before grilling or smoking to allow for absorption of flavor. For bigger cuts like brisket, it's best to apply seasoning the night before. Coat generously. You want a healthy amount of seasoning on every bite.

Don't be afraid to experiment. Dry rubs are an easy and forgiving way to develop your own style. A good dry rub not only seasons the meat but transforms it. That crusty, barky goodness you love on smoked ribs or brisket? All thanks to a dry rub.

[32]
BALANCING ACID, OIL, & HERBS IN WET MARINADES

While dry rubs make for a tasty exterior, marinades dive under the surface and into the meat. Consider marinades as magical potions that flavor and tenderize meat before it rides the grill.

THE FORMULA

Acid: Acid breaks down tough muscle fibers and tenderizes meat. Citrus, vinegar, wine, tomato juice, and yogurt are popular acids for marinades.

Oil: Oil locks moisture in and provides flavor deep inside the meat. Depending on what you're looking for, options include olive, canola, avocado, and sesame oil.

Flavorings: Garlic, ginger, soy sauce, chili, and mustard are popular. Plus, fresh herbs like basil, rosemary, and thyme are only a few of many options, so get creative!

BEST USES

Chicken and pork: These proteins benefit from marinades the most because they're leaner and will dry out quicker. A good soak keeps the meat juicy.

Beef: Marinades are great for tougher cuts of beef, like flank and skirt steak. Ribeye doesn't need a marinade, however, as marbling makes it naturally tender and flavorful.

Seafood: Marinades should only sit on seafood for thirty minutes, max. The last thing you want to do is wreck the delicate flakiness. Sometimes, less is best, and a good marinade will brighten this lean protein without tearing things apart.

PRO TIPS

Marinating isn't just about tenderness — it's about building layers. A soy-ginger marinade will add Asian inspiration to chicken thighs, while a red wine marinade gives beef a rich, deep flavor. Once you learn balance, you'll never have bland meat again. Follow these pro tips to level up your flavor:

- Don't go overboard with acid, or your meat will get mushy.
- Always marinate in the fridge; room-temperature marinating is an open invitation to bacteria.
- Use a sealed plastic bag or glass container, as acid can corrode metal.
- Pay attention to each oil's smoke point, especially if you're cooking with high heat.

[33]
HOMEMADE
BBQ SAUCES

Sauce is a vital part of any BBQ. It's the final ingredient that ties everything together. However, not all BBQ sauces are the same; the sheer number of regional varieties across America means that pitmasters can argue for hours as to which is the "real" BBQ sauce. Let's take a look at two of the most famous varieties: Kansas City and Carolina.

KANSAS CITY STYLE

This thick, sweet, and tangy sauce is what most people associate with BBQ. Tomato — typically ketchup — forms the base, which is then balanced with vinegar, molasses or brown sugar, and spices.

- **Flavor profile:** Sweet and smoky, with a hint of tang
- **Best on:** Ribs, chicken, and brisket
- **Pro tip:** Apply BBQ sauce in the last fifteen to twenty minutes of cooking to prevent the sugar from burning.

CAROLINA STYLE

Carolina BBQ is all about vinegar. This category of BBQ sauce is further divided into regional variations.

- **Eastern Carolina:** A thin, vinegar-based sauce finished with red pepper provides a tart contrast to the richness of pulled pork.
- **South Carolina:** Add mustard to the vinegar base to get a unique, tangy sauce with a hint of heat.
- **Flavor profile:** Tangy, sharp, and bright
- **Best on:** Pulled pork or whole-hog BBQ

WHY HOMEMADE IS BETTER THAN STORE-BOUGHT

Most sauces sold in stores are heavy on corn syrup and preservatives. Luckily, making your own sauce is easy and cheap, with endless options for customization. Besides, there's nothing more satisfying than the look on your guests' faces when you say, "Yeah, I made the sauce."

[34]
INJECTING MEATS
FOR DEEP FLAVOR

So now you know that dry rubs are great for outside seasoning, and marinades penetrate even deeper. However, when it comes to maximum flavor in every bite, injection is your best bet. As the term suggests, this method involves using a syringe-like tool to inject liquid seasoning directly into the meat.

Injections will help retain moisture in large cuts of meat, such as brisket, pork shoulder, and turkey, during long cooks. It also helps avoid the disappointment of a great bark concealing a bland interior.

HOW TO INJECT

- **Basic mix:** Broth (beef, chicken, or pork); melted butter; and a dash of salt
- **Beef:** Beef broth, Worcestershire sauce, garlic powder, and soy sauce
- **Pork:** Apple juice, cider vinegar, brown sugar, and a few dashes of hot sauce
- **Poultry:** Chicken stock, melted butter, lemon juice, and herbs

INJECTING

1. Fill the syringe with your preferred mixture.

2. Stick the needle deep into the meat, then slowly pull back while depressing the plunger.
3. Space the injections out about one inch apart for even coverage.

PRO TIPS

- Don't flood. Over-injecting creates pockets of liquid.
- Inject before applying rubs to seal in the flavor.
- Use a stainless-steel injector; plastic may be cheap, but it breaks easily.

Injecting is like an IV of flavor for your meat. Once you start using injectors, you'll never go back to surface-only seasoning!

[35]
WOOD TYPES
FOR SMOKING

In smoking, the wood you burn is just as important as the cut of meat or the rub you season it with. Similar to wine pairing, each type of wood imparts a different flavor, and finding the right variety is a game-changer. Wood isn't just a fuel source—it's an ingredient—so show it the same respect you would spices or sauces.

HICKORY

The classic wood for smoking, hickory produces strong, hearty, bacon-flavored smoke. It's best for pork shoulder, ribs, and beef brisket. However, hickory can become bitter, so use it as one wood in your balance of elements.

MESQUITE

A heavy lifter, mesquite burns hot and fast, with a bold, earthy flavor that can easily become overpowering if you're not careful.

It's best for beef (specifically steak and brisket). Use mesquite in moderation or mix with milder woods.

APPLE

The darling of smoking woods, applewood is mild, fruity, and sweet. It's best for poultry, pork, and seafood. Apple smoke works especially well when mixed with denser woods like oak.

OTHER COMMON OPTIONS

- **Cherry:** Sweet and colorful, imparts a nice dark-red coloring
- **Oak:** A medium-strength wood that can be used with almost any meat
- **Pecan:** Sweet and nutty, similar to some hickories but milder

[36]
CREATING YOUR
SIGNATURE SPICE BLEND

Almost every pit master envisions having a unique flavor associated with their BBQ, and blending spices is how you get there. Creating a signature seasoning is part science and part art.

Before you can achieve this feat, you'll need the building blocks:

- **Salt:** Kosher salt since it adheres to meat better and seasons more evenly
- **Sweet:** Brown sugar, white sugar, or even honey powder, which adds a caramelized look
- **Heat:** Black pepper, cayenne, chili flake, or hot paprika
- **Aromatics:** Garlic, onion, or mustard powder, cumin, etc.
- **Personality:** Smoked paprika, ground coffee, cinnamon, or dried herbs like rosemary and parsley

Now, follow these steps to create your very own mix:

1. **Start simple:** Experiment with ratios of basic ingredients: salt, pepper, paprika, and sugar.
2. **Experiment:** Once you have a baseline, start adding more exotic ingredients such as chili powder or coffee grounds, one or two at a time.
3. **Test:** Use small cuts of meat like chicken thighs to test. Make notes on flavor and balance.
4. **Refine:** Play with your mix until it practically screams *you*!

PRO TIPS

Consistency is key. Spice grinders are excellent tools to help create a uniform mix; you can also sift ingredients through a fine-mesh sieve. As you go along, make small batches for testing. Spices lose potency over time, so the fresher the blend, the better it will taste. Label *everything*. That way, if you hit the jackpot, you'll have the ratios written down.

EXAMPLE SIGNATURE BLENDS

Sweet and smoky pork rub: half a cup of brown sugar, a quarter cup of paprika, two tablespoons of salt, two tablespoons of black pepper, one tablespoon garlic powder, one tablespoon onion powder.

Bold beef rub: quarter cup kosher salt, two tablespoons black pepper, two tablespoons chili powder, one tablespoon cumin, one tablespoon ground coffee.

All-purpose blend: quarter cup salt, quarter cup paprika, two tablespoons garlic powder, two tablespoons onion powder, one tablespoon cayenne, one tablespoon thyme.

Your spice blend creates your signature flavor. Once you've created it, people will recognize your BBQ within the first bite.

[37]
GLAZES & MOPS
FOR BASTING

BBQ is also about how you manage flavor during the cook. That's where glazes and mops come into play.

MOPS

Mop sauce is a liquid, typically thin and vinegar-based, that's applied with a brush—or "mopped" on—during a long cook. The goal is to keep the surface of the meat moist, build layers of flavor, and provide a bright tang to balance richness.

- **Classic mop base:** Vinegar, water or stock, a bit of oil, and spices like chili flakes or black pepper
- **Best for:** Pork shoulders, ribs, and brisket—things you cook for hours on a smoker
- **Pro tip:** Mop lightly every hour or so. Drenching the meat will cool it down and lengthen cooking time.

GLAZES

Glazes are sticky, shiny concoctions brushed on meat near the end of cooking. Generally, glazes are thicker and sweeter than mops, and the sugar helps achieve that glossy finish we all love.

- **Classic glaze base:** Honey, molasses, or brown sugar; spices; fruit juice or vinegar
- **Best for:** Ribs, chicken wings, salmon
- **Pro tip:** Apply glazes within twenty to thirty minutes of serving to prevent burning the sugar.

[38]
PAIRING FLAVORS
WITH MEATS

Like any art, seasoning is all about balance. A rub that does wonders on pork ribs might overwhelm chicken or clash with fish. It's the combination of meat with the right flavor profile that distinguishes a pitmaster from a novice.

BEEF

Beef has a bold and rich flavor, so strong, earthy flavors are ideal.

- **Best pairings:** Black pepper, garlic, cumin, chili powder, coffee grounds
- **Woods:** Oak, mesquite, hickory
- **Sauces:** Peppery or tomato-based sauces with a nice smoky backbone

PORK

Pork is more versatile and likes a hint of sweetness and a crispy crust to offset its natural fatty flavor. Consequently, pork rubs lean to the sweet side but are second only to ribs smoked atop brown sugar. When matching flavors to meat, it's all about harmony.

- **Best pairings:** Brown sugar, paprika, apple, mustard, fennel
- **Woods:** Apple, cherry, pecan
- **Sauces:** Sweet or tangy glazes, Carolina mustard vinegar sauce

POULTRY

Chicken and turkey have milder flavor profiles, which basically provide a blank canvas for you to be as subtle or bold as you like.

- **Best pairings:** Lemon, rosemary, thyme, garlic, cayenne
- **Woods:** Apple, cherry, or pecan for lighter smoke

- **Sauces:** Citrus-based glazes, creamy white sauce, or light tomato-based sauces

SEAFOOD

Seafood has an even more delicate flavor, so restraint is definitely recommended.

- **Best pairings:** Dill, lemon, ginger, garlic, soy
- **Woods:** Alder, apple, cherry
- **Sauces:** Butter-based or soy-ginger glaze

[39]
COMMON FLAVOR MISTAKES

Mistakes happen, even to the best pitmasters. Flavor blunders can ruin hours of cooking, so let's address the big ones.

OVERSALTING

While salt is vital to any cook, it's all too easy to overdo it. Excessive salt can ruin even the best cut of meat with a harsh, bitter flavor. When using salt in a rub, apply lightly. You can always sprinkle more on later.

BURNING SUGAR

Burning sugar is another serious mistake to avoid. Caramelized sugar helps create a delicious crust, but go too far, and it turns into a bitter mess. Burned sugar usually makes an appearance when sauces or glazes are applied too early. It's best to only use sweet sauces in the last twenty minutes. Let the heat kiss it, not char it to death.

OVERDOING BLENDS

Loading up on every spice you can think of will create confusing results. In brisket, for example, less is often more. Use salt, pepper, garlic, and one or two strong flavor options rather than a twenty-spice jumble.

RELYING ON SAUCE

Sauce should help with flavor, not hide it. If you have to drown your meat in sauce just to make it palatable, something went wrong along the way, whether your rub, smoke, or time.

[40]
STORING & GIFTING
YOUR CUSTOM SAUCES

One of the most exciting aspects of BBQ is creating your very own sauce, allowing you to create an experience that's truly different and uniquely your own. Of course, once you perfect your signature flavor, it's time to think about preservation—and distribution.

STORING YOUR SAUCES

When it's time to store your sauces, clearly label each jar with the creation date as well as contents. There's nothing worse than trying to guess the contents of a mystery jar.

Short term: Store sauce in a tightly sealed jar or bottle; with refrigeration, most sauces keep for one to two weeks.

Long term: To create a bigger batch, properly can your product in sterilized jars. Vinegar-based sauces last the longest.

GIFTING YOUR SAUCES

Homemade sauce makes a great gift! Pack your sauce in mason jars or swing-top bottles and add a custom label for a present friends and family will actually use. Homemade sauces are perfect for occasions like Father's Day, birthdays, housewarming, or even a thank-you gift. Consider pairing your sauce with wood chips or a spice rub for an awesome BBQ gift pack.

CHAPTER FIVE: GRILLING TECHNIQUES

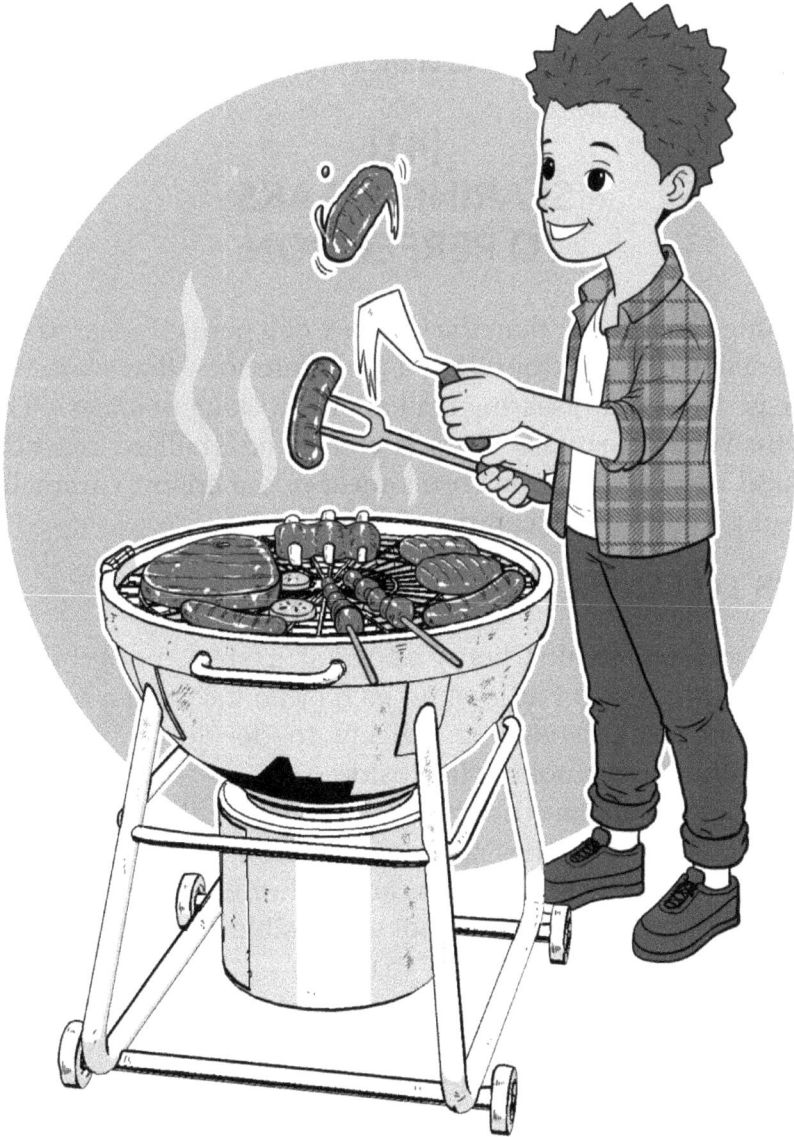

Grilling is all about what happens when fire and food meet. In this chapter, we will focus on fundamental grilling skills to take raw products to their smoky and delicious max. If you ever hear a grilling technique you're unsure about, this is the place to learn how to take your grilling game to the next level. From searing steaks to spatchcocking chickens, we will reveal all basic methods that truly define a casual griller and a pitmaster. Consider this your culinary guide to achieve the precision, timing, and flair needed so that every bite from your grill comes off as cooked to perfection.

[41]
SEARING STEAKS
TO PERFECTION

Few things are greater than the first bite of a perfectly seared steak. A delectable crust surrounding a juicy interior—that's where the magic is. To be clear, searing isn't about "locking in juices." That's a myth. What it actually does is create the Maillard reaction, a chemical process that transforms meat into a crispy, caramelized piece of goodness with complex flavors.

STEPS TO PERFECTLY SEAR

1. **Pick your steak:** Choose ribeye, strip steak, porterhouse, or sirloin. Aim for at least an inch or an inch and a half thick. Thin steaks cook too quickly to develop a good crust without overcooking the inside.
2. **Prepare the meat:** Pat the meat dry with paper towels. Moisture prevents the outside from browning. Season liberally with salt, pepper, and if desired, your rub.
3. **Heat it:** Get the grill as hot as possible. You want extreme, direct heat, around 500°F to 600°F.
4. **Sear both sides:** Once you place the steak, don't touch it for two to three minutes. Then flip the steak and leave it alone for another two to three minutes. Don't press down on it; that squeezes juice out.

5. **Finish to temperature:** After searing, transfer your steak to the indirect cooking zone until it reaches the desired doneness.

TIMING GUIDE

Here's a rough guide for a steak that's an inch and a half thick:

- **Rare (125°F):** Sear two to three minutes on each side, then cook two to three minutes indirectly.
- **Medium Rare (135°F):** Sear three to four minutes on each side, then cook three to five minutes indirectly.
- **Medium (145°F):** Sear four minutes on each side, then six to seven minutes indirectly.
- **Well done (160°F):** Honestly, don't... but if you must, just give it extra time on indirect heat.

PRO TIPS

- Always use a thermometer; winging it will leave you and your diners disappointed.
- Let your steaks rest for five to ten minutes after cooking to allow juices to redistribute.
- To get grill marks, rotate steaks 90° halfway through cooking each side.

A great sear is confidence on a plate. Once you master it, you will never again accept a bland, gray steak.

[42]
REVERSE SEARING
FOR THICK CUTS

With large cuts, such as tomahawks or two-inch ribeyes, searing first can burn the meat outside before it cooks on the inside. Enter reverse searing: smart cooking with more control. Instead of starting with direct heat, begin with indirect heat on low until the meat is almost done. Then finish by searing it hot. This way, you'll get an evenly cooked inside and a great crust.

THE STEPS

1. **Prepare the steak:** Use the standard method. Pat dry and season generously.
2. **Start low and slow:** Put the steak on the cool side of the grill (indirect heat) at about 225°F to 250°F until it reaches 10°F to 15°F below your target temperature. For a medium-rare steak (135°F), remove at 120°F.
3. **Rest for a few minutes:** Take the steak off the grill, then crank up the heat.
4. **Finish with fire:** Put the steak on for one or two minutes per side, quickly building a crust without worrying about cooking the inside.

TIMING GUIDE

Here's a guide for reverse searing a two-inch ribeye:

- **Rare (125°F):** Cook twenty to twenty-five minutes indirectly, then sear for two minutes.
- **Medium rare (135°F):** Cook twenty to twenty-five minutes indirectly, then sear for two to three minutes.
- **Medium (145°F):** Cook thirty to thirty-five minutes indirectly, then sear for three minutes.

If searing is power, reverse searing is finesse. Use it when you have a cut too thick for guesswork, and you'll look like a pro every time.

[43]
GRILLING BURGERS
WITHOUT SHRINKAGE

Burgers are the backbone of barbecue season, but all too often, we end up with shriveled pucks of despair that barely taste like beef. As ground beef cooks, it shrinks; when overworked or cooked too hot, it shrinks into thick, dry domes. The key to avoiding this involves handling, shaping, and cooking. As ground beef cooks, it shrinks; when overworked or cooked too hot, it shrinks into thick, dry domes.

THE GUIDE TO THE PERFECT BURGER

1. **Choose the right ground beef:** Settle on eighty percent lean and twenty percent fat. Too lean, and the burger will be dry; too fatty, and the burger will be a greasy mess.
2. **Gentle patties:** Make patties up to an inch thick. Don't overwork, or it'll get tough.
3. **Indent the patties:** Using your thumb, create an indentation in the middle of each patty to help prevent "doming."
4. **Keep seasoning simple:** Add salt and pepper right before you hit the grill to prevent the salt from drawing moisture out of the beef.
5. **Grill hot and fast:** Direct heat at around 450°F to 500°F is ideal. Cook for three to five minutes per side, depending on your preference.
6. **Don't smash the patties:** Pressing down with a spatula squeezes juice and flavor out of the burger.

TIMING GUIDE

Here's a timing guide for three-quarter-inch patties:

- **Medium rare (135°F):** Cook three minutes per side.
- **Medium (145°F):** Cook four minutes per side.
- **Well done (160°F):** Cook five minutes per side.

PRO TIPS

- Add cheese during the last minute of cooking, then cover the grill to melt the cheese.
- To add a pro touch, toast buns for thirty seconds right before assembling burgers.
- Allow burgers to rest for two minutes before serving to retain juices.

[44]
KEBAB & SKEWER ASSEMBLY

Kebabs are not only a fun crowd-pleaser; they're also adaptable and easy to eat. Kebabs are the finger-food of BBQ: accessible, adaptable, and perfect for showcasing your culinary creativity.

Of course, kebabs also have the potential for uneven cooking—with charred vegetables and undercooked meat or, conversely, dry meat and raw veggies. Ultimately, the key to a successful kebob comes down to assembly and balance.

CHOOSING SKEWERS

Metal skewers conduct heat and, therefore, cook meat from the inside out, which is a big point in their favor. Wood skewers are fine, but soaking them for thirty minutes before grilling will help avoid flare-ups. When possible, use flat skewers to prevent food from spinning when you turn them.

ASSEMBLING

- **Same size:** Cut your meat and vegetables into regular pieces so that they cook at the same rate.
- **Separate skewers:** Instead of cooking meat and vegetables together, put them on separate skewers for more controlled cooking.
- **Mind the gaps:** Leave space between each piece; crowded skewers prevent heat from circulating evenly.
- **Balance the fat:** Alternate fat (e.g., chicken thighs) with lighter vegetables (e.g., peppers).

COOKING

Cook kebabs on a medium-high grill, turning every few minutes. Most meat skewers cook in ten to twelve minutes, while veggie skewers only take about six to eight minutes. Maintain moisture by basting with oil before cooking or applying a light glaze.

[45]
WHOLE CHICKEN
SPATCHCOCKING

Grilling a whole chicken may be dazzling, but it can also be a challenge. Without the right methods, you could end up with dry breast meat and raw thighs. Never fear—spatchcocking is here! This prep method turns a whole bird into a flat piece of meat that will cook evenly on the grill.

Spatchcocking, or "butterflying," involves taking the back off a chicken and flattening it to put it on the grill. Having all parts of the bird in contact with heat allows for faster, more even cooking and provides a beautiful presentation.

SPATCHCOCK CHICKEN

1. **Get sharp shears:** Turn the chicken breast-side down and cut along both sides of the backbone, then remove the backbone completely.
2. **Flatten it:** Flip the chicken breast-side up. Press down firmly on the breastbone until it cracks, allowing the chicken to lie flat.
3. **Season:** Pat the skin dry with paper towels, then rub with oil, salt, pepper, and your choice of seasoning blend.

FOR GRILLING A SPATCHCOCK CHICKEN

1. **Heat:** Apply indirect heat at roughly 375°F to 400°F. Put your chicken skin-side up on the cooler side of the grill.
2. **Cooking time:** Cook for approximately forty-five to sixty minutes, depending on the size of your chicken. The internal temperature of the breast should be 165°F and 175°F at the thighs.

3. **Finishing move:** Flip the chicken skin-side down over direct heat for two to three minutes to crisp up the skin before serving.

PRO TIPS

- Save the backbone to make stock. It's liquid gold.
- To add flavor, marinate or brine the chicken before grilling.
- For subtle smoke, throw a few chips of applewood or pecan on the hot coals.

[46]
VEGGIE GRILLING
WITHOUT CHARRING

Vegetables shouldn't be an afterthought at a BBQ. Grill with skill, and both vegan and omnivorous guests will fill their plates with grilled veggies. When grilled correctly, veggies add sweetness, color, and balance to smoky meats. When grilled poorly, on the other hand, they become charred, inedible husks that nobody wants to see, let alone eat.

As long as you choose wisely, prep correctly, and stick with lower temps, grilled veggies will be a great addition to your BBQ repertoire. Peppers, zucchini, eggplant, mushrooms, corn, and asparagus are great for grilling. Leafy greens and overly soft vegetables don't do well over open flame.

PREP TIPS

- **Slice wisely:** Start by cutting your veggies into large, uniform pieces. Thinly sliced veggies tend to burn quickly.
- **Use oil sparingly:** Oiling helps your veggies brown and caramelize, but use a brush, not a bottle. Dripping grease can cause flare-ups.
- **Season simply:** Stick to salt, pepper, garlic, and herbs—no need to get carried away.

COOKING TECHNIQUES

Veggies like asparagus, zucchini, and mushrooms can be grilled directly on the grates for three to five minutes, turning occasionally. For denser veggies like corn on the cob and whole bell peppers, cook indirectly for about fifteen to twenty minutes. If you're cooking smaller veggies, use a grill basket to keep them from falling through the grates.

PRO TIPS

- Add a squeeze of lemon juice after grilling for brightness and acidity.
- Don't overcook; vegetables should be tender but retain some crunch.
- If you're feeling fancy, finish with a drizzle of balsamic glaze or sprinkle with fresh parmesan cheese.

[47]
PIZZA ON THE GRILL

Believe it or not, your grill can be a pizza oven. Done right, grilled pizza is smoky, crisp, and better than delivery. However, it takes a little finesse to get it right.

THE DOUGH

- **Homemade:** Dough is just a mixture of flour, yeast, water, salt, and olive oil. Let it rise until it doubles in size, then stretch it out to thin.
- **Store-bought:** There's no shame in using a store-bought dough! It works just as well on the grill.

HOW TO GRILL PIZZA

1. **Get your grill hot:** Aim for about 500°F. You want direct heat to crisp your dough.

2. **Oil your dough:** Lightly brush olive oil on both sides to prevent sticking.
3. **Grill first side:** Lay your stretched dough directly over the grill grates. Grill for two to three minutes until you see bubbles and char marks forming.
4. **Flip and top:** Once you've grilled your first side, flip the dough and quickly add sauce, cheese, and toppings.
5. **Finish with lid closed:** Close your grill for three to five minutes to melt the cheese and cook the pizza all the way through.

SOME IDEAS FOR TOPPINGS

- **Margherita:** Tomato, fresh mozzarella, basil
- **Meat lovers:** Pepperoni, sausage, pulled pork
- **BBQ:** BBQ sauce, grilled chicken, red onion, cilantro

[48]
FOIL PACKETS
FOR EASY SIDES

Sides often don't get as much attention on BBQs as they deserve, but they play a key role in completing your meal. Foil packets allow you to multitask. Just set up the grill, put your meal on, and let the sides do their thing.

Foil packets work by holding in steam while providing moisture to food. They also keep small food items (like diced potatoes and shrimp) from falling through the grates. Plus, they're easy to clean up. Just toss the foil when you're finished.

HOW TO MAKE A FOIL PACKET

1. Lay out a sheet of heavy-duty foil.
2. Wrap ingredients in the foil.
3. Don't be shy with seasoning. Use plenty of salt, pepper, and spices.

4. Seal the foil tightly by folding edges over to prevent steam from escaping.
5. Place over indirect heat and grill until food is fully cooked, generally twenty to thirty minutes, depending on your ingredients.

GREAT COMBINATIONS

- Potato and onion with butter, garlic, and rosemary
- Shrimp boil with shrimp, corn, sausage, potatoes, and Cajun seasoning
- Veggie medley of zucchini, mushrooms, peppers, and balsamic glaze

[49]
RESTING MEAT

One misstep beginners often make is taking meat off the grill and then immediately slicing into it. The result: juice all over the plate and none in your meat. During cooking, heat pushes juices to the center of the meat. Resting allows the juices to redistribute evenly throughout the cut. If you skip this step, you'll lose a lot of moisture and flavor.

HOW LONG TO REST

- **Steak and chops:** Five to ten minutes
- **Roasts and brisket:** Twenty to thirty minutes or up to an hour if wrapped in foil and towels
- **Poultry:** Fifteen to twenty minutes for a whole bird

PRO TIPS

- Tent loosely in foil to keep warm, but don't wrap too tightly or steam will ruin the crust.
- Use a cutting board with a juice groove. Resting will release some liquid, and you don't want a waterfall on your counter.

[50]
CARVING
LIKE A BOSS

Considering you've mastered cooking, let's not overlook presentation. How you carve your meat has an impact on tenderness, so it might cost you if you don't do it properly. The number one rule is to cut across the grain. Muscle fibers are arranged in one direction. When you cut across them, you shorten them, making the meat tender. Cut with the grain and you're probably going to have chewy meat.

CARVING METHODS

- **Brisket:** Separate the point from the flat, then slice across the grain into quarter-inch slices.
- **Steaks:** If you're going to slice your steaks, cut thin slices against the grain.
- **Poultry:** For a whole chicken or turkey, remove the legs, thighs, and wings. Then carve the breast meat into slices.
- **Ribs:** Cut between the bones with a sharp knife. If you have a lot of bark, make sure to keep it intact.

Pro Tips

- Use a long, sharp carving knife.
- Keep slices even for a professional presentation.
- Warm plates in advance. Cold surfaces will sap heat, leaving you with cold meat.

Carving isn't just cutting; it's the final act of the BBQ show. When done correctly, carving gives your meal that final touch to ensure your food looks as good as it tastes.

CHAPTER SIX:
SMOKING &
LOW-AND-SLOW MAGIC

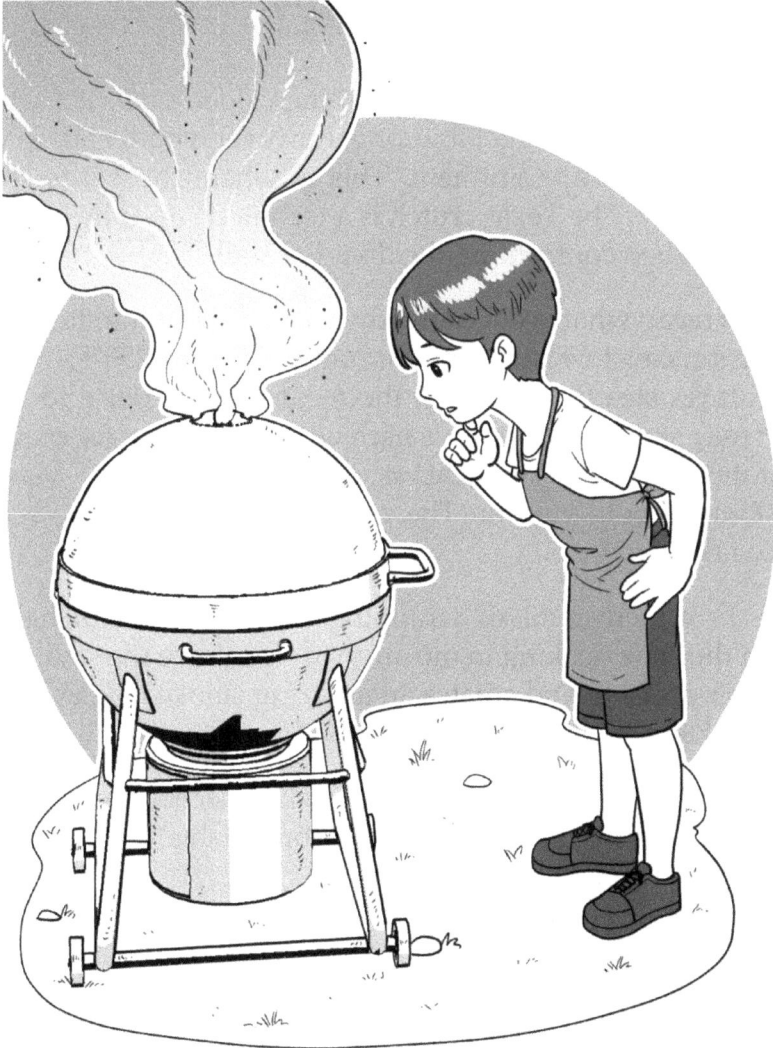

While grilling is essentially fast and furious, smoking is slow and deliberate. Low-and-slow cooking transforms tough cuts into smoky perfection. Here, you'll get the lowdown on three methods: Texas crutch for brisket, rib methods (3-2-1 vs. straight smoke), and the secret to perfect pulled pork.

[51]
THE TEXAS CRUTCH
FOR BRISKET

Brisket is the crown jewel of BBQ. When done well, it's tender, smoky, and juicy. If you get it wrong, however, you'll end up with a dry, leathery disappointment. This is where the Texas crutch comes into play. The Texas crutch is a technique used by barbecue pitmasters when confronting the dreaded stall.

First, let's recap what you've already learned about the stall. When smoking brisket low and slow, around 225°F to 250°F, internal temperatures steadily rise until the meat reaches 150°F to 160°F. Then it may stall for hours. This happens because surface moisture evaporates, cooling the meat as it cooks—the same way air conditioning cools a room. The resulting stall can make a cook seem to take forever.

The Texas crutch involves wrapping the brisket about halfway through the cook, locking in moisture to rise above the stall. It also accelerates cooking and creates an amazing smoke ring even with the wrap. Here's how to use this method:

1. Smoke, unwrapped, until the brisket reaches about 160°F.
2. Wrap tightly in butcher paper (breathable) or heavy-duty foil (for moisture retention).
3. Continue cooking until internal temp reaches 200°F to 205°F.
4. Rest for at least an hour before slicing.

PRO TIP

Paper maintains texture integrity, giving you a better bark. Meanwhile, foil retains more moisture. Depending on your priorities, use whichever you prefer. The Texas crutch is a game-changer, especially if you're new to brisket. It eliminates some of the guesswork, giving you consistency and confidence.

[52]
RIB METHODS

Ribs are definitely the star of BBQ, but pitmasters are divided on the best way to cook them. The two main contenders are the 3-2-1 method and straight smoke. The 3-2-1 method is great for novice pitmasters looking to create fall-off-the-bone ribs. It's easily summarized in three steps:

1. **3 hours of smoke:** Cook ribs uncovered at 225°F and let them absorb smoke.
2. **2 hours wrapped:** Next, wrap in foil with a bit of apple juice, butter, or sauce to braise.
3. **1-hour post-glaze:** Unwrap and sauce the ribs, then return to the smoker to set the glaze.

This method is tough to mess up. The ribs will be tender with consistent results. However, some pitmasters argue that this method results in overcooking.

STRAIGHT SMOKE

This is the traditional technique. Smoke the ribs, unwrapped, at 225°F to 250°F until done. It usually takes five to six hours, so the cook time is comparable to the 3-2-1 method. If you follow this school of thought, you'll have smoke, bark, and meat that pulls cleanly from the bone without falling apart. The downside is that it isn't forgiving, so if you mistime it, then your ribs will dry out.

WHICH IS BETTER?

If you're cooking for a backyard BBQ with family and friends, the 3-2-1 method is probably the way to go. If you're competing or you simply want ribs with true bite, then straight smoke is the better choice.

You can always try a hybrid. Smoke the ribs unwrapped for four hours, then finish with a short wrap—around thirty minutes—to maintain that moist, juicy texture. Both of these techniques have their time and place. Ultimately, the true winner is whichever method fits your personality and palate.

[53]
PULLED PORK
SECRETS

Pulled pork is the ultimate BBQ comfort food: smoky, juicy, melt-in-your-mouth shreds of pork shoulder (Boston butt). But to get it right, you'll need to be patient and know a few tricks. The first step is choosing the right cut. When selecting your pork shoulder, look for marbling and a fat cap. A pork shoulder typically weighs between six and ten pounds—a perfect size to feed a group.

THE PROCESS

1. **Prep:** Remove excess fat, leaving a quarter-inch cap. Rub spice mix (paprika, sugar, garlic, cayenne) liberally over the pork.
2. **Low and slow:** Smoke at 225°F to 250°F with the wood of your choice (hickory, apple, pecan).
3. **The stall:** Like brisket, pork shoulder stalls around 160°F. You can either ride it out or use the Texas crutch by wrapping it in foil or butcher paper.
4. **Finish temp:** Cook until the internal temperature reaches approximately 203°F. It should be like soft butter.

5. **Rest:** Rest for at least one hour in a cooler or bundled in towels.
6. **Shred it:** Shred your pork with meat claws or a couple of forks, then toss with reserved juices or a splash of vinegar sauce to keep it moist.

PRO TIPS

- Spritz the pork during the process with apple juice or apple cider vinegar to maintain moisture in the bark.
- Don't skimp on resting! Rested pork will pull cleaner and maintain its juiciness.
- Serve with buns, coleslaw, and pickles for a killer sandwich.

[54]
COLD SMOKING
CHEESES & NUTS

When people think about smoking, they usually envision ribs or brisket. However, smoking can add a terrific flavor to foods you may never have considered smoking, like cheese and nuts. Cold smoking is the best method for this.

Cold smoking happens at temperatures between 70°F and 90°F. It adds flavor without actually cooking the food. Because it doesn't involve heat, it's perfect for delicate food items like cheese, nuts, and even butter or salt.

COLD SMOKING CHEESE

1. **Choose the right cheese:** Hard cheeses like cheddar, Gouda, and mozzarella are the best candidates for smoking. Avoid using soft cheeses, which will melt too quickly.
2. **Prep:** Cut cheese into blocks and set on a wire rack. Let it sit at room temperature for one hour to develop a dry skin (or *pellicle*).

3. **Smoke source:** Use either a smoke tube or pellet maze, but don't put cheese over direct fire. You want thin, clean smoke, not flames.
4. **Time:** Cold smoke for two to four hours, flipping halfway through.
5. **Rest:** Wrap in parchment or vacuum seal the cheese, then rest in the fridge for one week. This allows the smoke to mellow and balance.

COLD SMOKING NUTS

1. **Spread:** Spread out almonds, pecans, or cashews on a tray.
2. **Smoke:** Cold smoke for one to two hours using apple or pecan woods.
3. **Toss:** After smoking, toss nuts with butter and seasoning for an amazing snack.

PRO TIPS

- Cold smoking is best at temperatures below 70°F.
- Always monitor your temperature; if it gets too hot, your cheese will become fondue.
- Smoked cheese is an amazing addition to burgers, mac and cheese, and charcuterie boards.

[55]
MAINTAINING TEMPERATURE IN SMOKERS

If BBQ has one rule, this is it: *Consistency is king.* Maintaining control of the temperature is critically important. Meat needs consistent heat to break down collagen and fat. Steady temperatures also mean predictable cook times.

Don't trust the cheap dial built into your smoker's lid. Invest in a digital probe thermometer to read both the meat and ambient temperature. You'll also need to check your airflow. More air equals a hotter fire. If you're worried about drying out your meat, use a water pan to improve stability and add moisture.

FUEL MANAGEMENT

Charcoal smokers: Add fuel slowly and steadily throughout the cook. Use a chimney starter to have hot coals ready to go when you need them.

Wood smokers: For even burning, cleaner smoke, and consistent temperature, always use seasoned wood splits, not green wood.

Pellet smokers: The beauty of pellets is that they're self-regulating. Just keep them dry and topped up.

TACTICS FOR MAINTAINING STABILITY

1. Always preheat your smoker before adding meat — *always*.
2. Only make small changes. If you over-correct, your temperatures will swing everywhere.
3. Don't lift the lid too often; you lose heat and smoke every time.

[56]
FORMING BARK

When someone bites into your brisket or ribs, the bark is the first layer they see and taste. Bark is that dark, crusty layer surrounding smoked meat that BBQ enthusiasts love — smoky, salty, and savory, with incredible flavor. However, bark isn't just created by chance; it's the direct result of chemistry, seasoning, and patience.

The rub determines the bark. The salt, sugar, spices, and herbs combine with juices to form a sticky paste. As the paste dries, it traps smoke molecules. Over time, amino acids and sugars caramelize, creating complex flavors that develop into the desired crust.

HOW TO BUILD GREAT BARK

1. **Use excess rub:** Don't be shy! Use a thick layer of rub so that there's plenty of substance to caramelize.
2. **Low and slow:** A good bark develops best in a long-cook environment of 225°F to 250°F. Too hot, and the sugar will burn; too cool, and the rub may not set up.
3. **Be careful with spritzing:** You can use apple cider vinegar or juice to keep the surface tacky, but don't drown it. Too much moisture will wash the bark away.
4. **Avoid foil too early:** Wrapping before the bark develops softens the bark. If you're using the Texas crutch, make sure the crust is solid before you wrap it.

COMMON MISTAKES

- **Sugar burn:** If you use too much sugar at high temperatures, it will burn, leading to bitter bark.
- **Weak smoke:** Thin blue smoke provides flavor, while thick white smoke drowns the meat and ruins the bark.
- **Impatience:** Bark doesn't develop in minutes but in hours. Rushing results in a soft crust.

PRO TIP

- Experiment with a variety of woods. Hickory produces a bolder piece of meat, while applewood imparts a sweeter tone.

[57]
THE SMOKE RING

One of the most sought-after characteristics of a perfectly smoked piece of meat is the thin pink layer just beneath the surface, which we call a smoke ring. Pitmasters proudly display their smoke ring as a badge of honor, and while it may seem like BBQ magic, it's simply science at work.

A smoke ring is formed when the gases from burning wood or charcoal, most commonly nitrogen dioxide, are combined with the meat's natural myoglobin. During low-and-slow cooking, the gases penetrate the meat and don't allow it to turn fully brown on the exterior. This leaves a thin pink layer that adds to the beauty of smoked brisket or ribs, as well as making it seem like an artistic expression.

The smoke ring does not add flavor by itself; however, it reveals a technique and lots of factors involved in establishing a steady fire, burning clean fuel, seasoning the wood, and proper airflow. All of these contribute to achieving a smoke ring. Once you have a smoke ring, you have proven to yourself that you successfully managed the fire and can officially call yourself a pitmaster.

[58]
JERKY MAKING
AT HOME

Jerky isn't just a snack from your local gas station; it's one of mankind's oldest methods of preserving food. David Dawson improved jerky by smoking it. When you do it yourself at home, you control the flavor, salt, and texture.

Lean cuts are best for making jerky. Look for beef top round, eye of round, flank steak, or venison. Don't use fatty cuts, as fat goes rancid in storage.

THE STEPS

1. **Slice thin:** Always slice against the grain in eighth-inch to quarter-inch strips. Cooling the meat slightly helps cut strips more easily.
2. **Marinate:** Common ingredients include soy sauce, Worcestershire sauce, garlic, onion, brown sugar, and spices. Marinate in the fridge for at least six hours—overnight is even better.

3. **Dry:** Smoke with a preheater smoker at around 160°F to180°F. Run strips across racks without overlapping too much, then smoke for three to five hours. Jerky should be chewy, not brittle.
4. **Store:** Store in airtight bags or jars and refrigerate for long-term storage.

PRO TIPS

- Add chili flakes or cayenne when marinating for extra heat.
- Experiment with different woods; applewood is sweet, while hickory is punchy.
- Rotate racks if your smoker has hot spots.

[59]
SMOKING SALMON
FOR BREAKFAST BBQS

BBQ isn't just for dinner. Smoked salmon can also create an unforgettable morning BBQ, whether on a bagel, scrambled with eggs, or served with cream cheese.

HOT VS. COLD

Hot-smoked salmon: Smoke at 225°F until flaky and fully cooked (approximately 145°F internal). This offers a bold taste that's perfect for cooking.

Cold-smoked salmon: After curing the fish with salt and sugar, smoke at 70°F to 80°F. The result is a delicate, silky flavor. Think lox on a bagel.

HOT SMOKING

1. **Brine:** In a bowl, mix water, kosher salt, and brown sugar, then brine salmon fillets for six to eight hours.

2. **Dry:** After brining, pat dry and let sit uncovered in the refrigerator for one to two hours to create a pellicle, the tacky surface that smoke clings to.
3. **Smoke:** When you're ready, smoke at 225°F for two to three hours until the fish reaches an internal temperature of 145°F. Fruit woods like apple, alder, or cherry work well with salmon.
4. **Serve:** Eat it right off the cutting board, over scrambled eggs, or add to salads.

PRO TIP

- Always use skin-on fillets; skin holds the salmon together for easy handling.

[60]
OVERNIGHT SMOKING

Successful overnight cooks are one of the most significant aspects of dedication in the barbecue world. Brisket, pork shoulder, and most other large cuts of meat are going to take anywhere from 10 to 16 hours on the smoker, which means that you're going to have to have the fire steady for quite some time after you head to bed. It may seem a little daunting, but if you prepare properly and put some checks into action, you'll be able to execute an overnight smoke without too much loss of sleep.

The key is proper setup for consistency before you even start. Use a quality smoker designed to hold heat, and the best fuel that will burn slowly, such as briquettes or hardwood chunks. Fill your water pan, check all the vents, and establish an appropriate temperature in the range of 225 to 250°F. Many pitmasters invest in wireless thermometers with alarms so they can lie in bed until something goes off.

Where and how you position your equipment is also vitally important. Your smoker should be set up in a safe spot, not exposing it to wind or combustible materials, and always have a fire extinguisher close by. Some people actually light the fire at night so that they can have a lunch selection ready for the next day.

The notion behind overnight smoking is always trust, trust that your smoker is properly set, trust in your fuel supply, and above all, trust that your patience will pay off. If you're fortunate enough to get that notion right, when you wake up in the morning, you will be met with a smell that is nearly to the realm of perfection.

CHAPTER SEVEN:
SIDES, SALADS, & EXTRAS

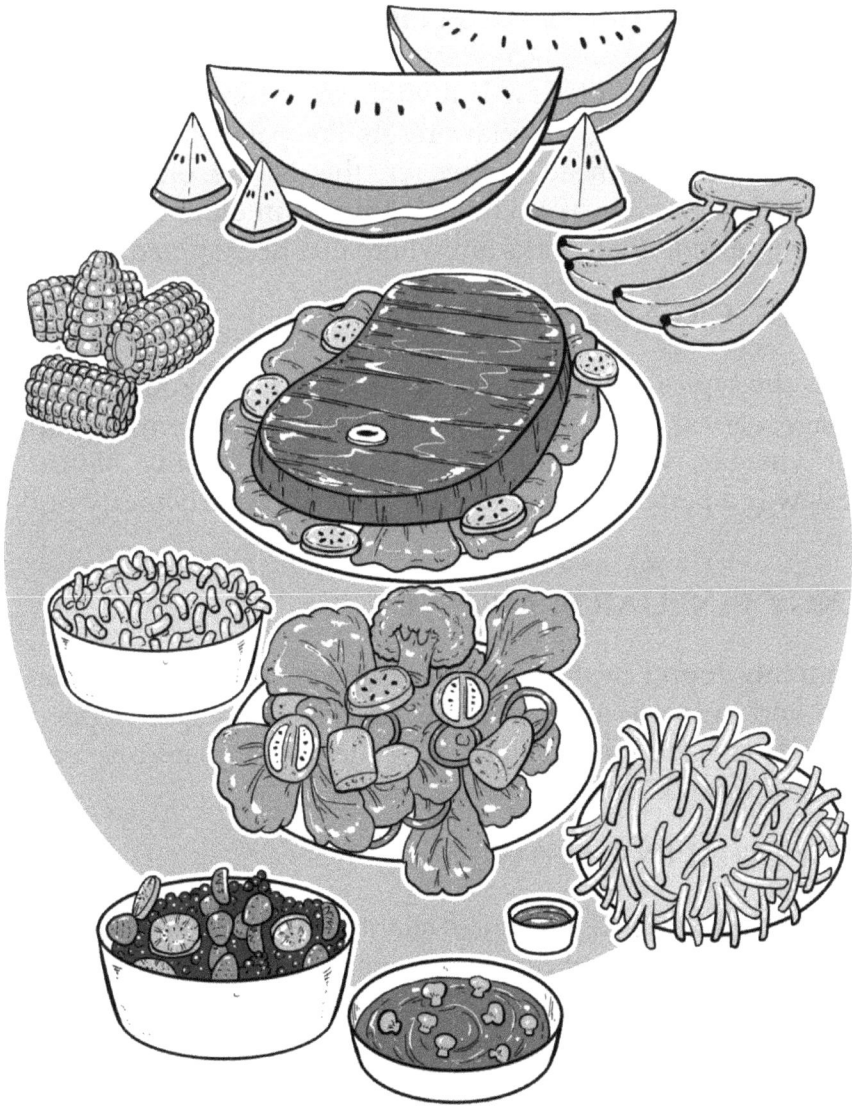

A real BBQ feast is about the whole plate. Sides provide fresh balance to the richness of your meat, and a spectacular side may even outshine the main course.

[61]
CLASSIC COLESLAW VARIATIONS

No doubt about it: coleslaw is a vital part of any BBQ. Crunchy, tangy, and refreshing, coleslaw resets the palate after the dense flavors of smoked meats. However, this isn't a one-size-fits-all dish. With a few tweaks, you can transform slaw into a multi-dimensional side that works anywhere in a BBQ spread.

CLASSIC CREAMY SLAW

This is the typical slaw found at any backyard cookout: shredded cabbage, carrots, and onions tossed in a dressing of mayo, apple cider vinegar, sugar, and celery seed. The creamy nature of coleslaw is a perfect companion for spicy BBQ, particularly pulled pork.

TANGY VINEGAR SLAW

Commonly found in the Carolinas, vinegar slaw lacks the fat of mayo and, instead, leans into the acidity of vinegar, sugar, and mustard. This slaw has a light, crisp flavor compared to creamy slaw, and it holds up better on sandwiches.

SPICY JALAPEÑO SLAW

The addition of sliced jalapeños, cilantro, and lime juice creates a spicy, crunchy slaw that can complement tacos, grilled chicken, or brisket.

PRO TIPS

- Shred cabbage very thinly; no matter how rugged and well thought-out the recipe, heavy chunks make for a clunky slaw.
- Let the slaw sit in the fridge for a minimum of one hour before you serve it. In fact, marinating overnight can bring flavors out in a way that even the freshest ingredients can't deliver.
- Include purple cabbage and mix in colorful vegetables for aesthetic perfection.

[62]
GRILLED CORN
ON THE COB HACKS

Nothing says "summer BBQ" like corn on the cob. It's simple, harkens to childhood, and can be topped with just about any flavor. Consequently, real pitmasters keep a couple of tricks up their sleeves to take plain corn to the next level.

Grilling in husk: Soak ears for thirty minutes, then grill. The husks steam corn, keeping it juicy. When done, pull back the husks and char them for some smoky flavor.

Grilling naked: For more flavor, remove husks and throw ears straight on the grill to caramelize the kernels.

FLAVOR HACKS

Grilled corn is the embodiment of a simple yet epic side. With the right hack, grilled corn has the potential to outdo the main meat.

- **Traditional butter and salt:** Keep it simple. Brush melted butter on the corn and sprinkle with sea salt.
- **Mexican street corn (elote):** Spread warm corn with mayo, then sprinkle with cotija cheese and chili powder. Next,

squeeze on some lime juice. The result is rich, messy, and delicious.

- **Garlic-parmesan corn:** Add butter, garlic, and parmesan cheese for upscale, savory flavor.
- **Bacon-wrapped corn:** Wrap ears in bacon, then grill. You'll be basting the corn in rich, flavorful fat while the bacon crisps.

PRO TIPS

- Use a skewer or corn holder for easy handling.
- Roll corn ears in flavored butter (herb, chipotle, honey) just before serving.
- When making large batches, keep grilled corn warm in a towel-lined cooler.

[63]
BAKED BEANS
WITH A TWIST

No BBQ spread is complete without baked beans. Smoky and sweet, hearty and filling, this side finishes off the meal and mops up BBQ sauce like a pro. Forget canned, syrupy beans. Homemade baked beans are the way to go. Do it right, and your guests will be reaching for seconds before they even think of brisket.

BASE & SAUCE

For the base, both navy beans and pinto beans work fine. Soak overnight, then cook the following day until tender. You can use canned beans if you prefer; just remember to drain and rinse them first.

Next, it's time to think about the sauce. In its most basic and traditional form, sauce is made with a combination of ketchup, molasses, brown sugar, mustard, and Worcestershire. These aren't

86

bad ingredients, but BBQ is all about bold flavors, so don't be afraid to play with them. Here are a few fun twists:

- **Bacon and onion beans:** First, cook bacon to render fat, then sauté onions in that fat and stir them into beans to add depth and smokiness to your beans.
- **Whiskey-infused beans:** A splash of bourbon or whiskey adds rich flavor and complexity.
- **Spicy BBQ beans:** Jalapeños, chipotle peppers, and hot sauce are excellent additions to baked beans.
- **Pulled pork beans:** Stir in leftover pulled pork for ramped-up flavor and texture.

THE PROCESS

Smoker method: Place beans in a cast iron skillet or dutch oven. Set the temperature at 225°F to 250°F and smoke for two to three hours. Stir occasionally to obtain an even flavor.

Oven shortcut: When the smoker is full and you're running out of time to get this done, you can bake beans in the oven at 300°F for one to two hours.

PRO TIPS

- If your beans are drying out, a small splash of apple juice or beer should freshen them up in a jiffy.
- Adding shredded cheese or breadcrumbs just before the finish will create a nice, crusty topping.

[64]
POTATO SALADS
THAT IMPRESS

While potato salad has been around forever, too often, it arrives bland, mushy, and drowning in mayo. However, that doesn't mean your potato salad can't be a showstopper! Read on to learn how this side can elevate BBQ rather than diminish it.

THE CREAMY CLASSIC

Use Yukon gold or red potatoes, which hold their shape better than starchy russets. Boil until just tender, not mushy, then toss with mayo, mustard, celery, onions, and diced hard-boiled eggs.

GERMAN-STYLE POTATO SALAD

This warm, tangy salad is a mayo-free option. Toss diced potatoes with vinegar, Dijon mustard, bacon, and onions. The result is a bold, smoky side that cuts rich BBQ as only potato salad can.

RANCH POTATO SALAD

Toss potatoes with ranch dressing, shredded cheddar cheese, and chives. Add crumbled bacon for a little more bang. This variety is like BBQ on a loaded baked potato.

SPICY CHIPOTLE POTATO SALAD

If you like it hot, blend chipotle peppers in adobo with either mayo or sour cream until smooth. Toss with potatoes, corn, and cilantro. This version provides smoky spice to the plate without overpowering the BBQ.

EXTRA SUGGESTIONS

- Salt the water liberally when boiling potatoes to season from the inside out.
- Creamy potato salads benefit from being chilled for at least two hours before serving.
- Use an assortment of red and purple potatoes for an eye-catching presentation.

[65]
BREAD & BUNS—
GRILLING THEM RIGHT

You can spend hours perfecting your brisket or pulled pork, but if you just throw it on a flimsy, frozen bun, you've just wasted half the work you put in. Bread and buns are worth the effort, too. They're the base of every BBQ sandwich or side bite.

Grilling bread adds a smoky flavor, lovely crunch, and a warm base to elevate BBQ, which is a huge win in any book. Even a quick char can elevate run-of-the-mill buns to something truly special.

- **Buns:** Brioche, potato rolls, or pretzel buns for pulled pork and burgers
- **Loaf:** Ciabatta, sourdough, or French bread for slicing and toasting
- **Flatbreads:** Pita or naan for quick-grilled bites to pair with BBQ

TECHNIQUES

Direct heat toasting: Place cut-side down over medium heat for thirty to sixty seconds. Watch for golden edges. Pay attention to timing, and don't let the crust blacken.

Garlic-butter brush: For a more indulgent option, mix garlic and herbs with butter before brushing it on the bread. It's impossible to resist grilled bread brushed with garlic and herbs.

Cheesy pull-apart bread: Want to mix things up? Slice your loaf into a grid without cutting all the way through. Stuff each slot with cheese and herbs, then wrap in foil and warm on the grill until the cheese melts.

PRO TIPS

- Always toast buns last at the very end, right before serving, or they'll dry out.
- Have a foil tray on hand to keep finished bread warm.
- Brush your buns with bacon fat instead of butter to see some barbecue magic.

[66]
PICKLES & RELISHES
FROM SCRATCH

BBQ is inherently rich, smoky, and heavy. This is where acidity plays its role. Pickles and relishes offer a sharp counterbalance to the fattiness of BBQ, rejuvenate the palate, and add a satisfying crunch. Store-bought options are fine in a pinch, but scratch-made immediately elevates your BBQ spread.

QUICK REFRIGERATOR PICKLES

You don't need weeks of fermentation to get fantastic flavor.

1. Slice cucumbers, onions, or jalapeños and place in jars (or another suitable container).
2. Boil vinegar, water, sugar, salt, and spices. Mustard seed, dill, and garlic are good options.
3. Pour the mixture over your sliced veggies in jars or containers.
4. Chill for twenty-four hours before eating.

Pickles will stay good and crispy in the fridge for two to three weeks.

TRADITIONAL DILL PICKLES

For a simple fermented version, pack cucumbers in salt brine with dill, garlic, and spices. Leave them to ferment at room temperature for five to seven days, then refrigerate for a garlicky, tangy treat.

BBQ RELISHES

- **Corn relish:** Fill a jar with sweet corn kernels, peppers, onions, and vinegar for a colorful, zesty condiment.
- **Spicy pepper relish:** A combination of roasted peppers, vinegar, and sugar makes a subtly sweet condiment with a hint of heat.

PRO TIPS

- The idea is to balance sweet, salty, and sour in a cohesive whole without overpowering your meal.
- Don't limit yourself to cucumbers! Try pickling carrots, green beans, or even watermelon rind.
- Use non-reactive containers whenever you're working with vinegar: glass and stainless-steel work best.

[67]
FRUIT ON THE GRILL

Grilled fruit may seem odd to some, but it's a barbecue staple. Heat caramelizes natural sugars, yielding a flavor that's both smoky and sweet, indulgent yet refreshing.

PINEAPPLE

Grilled pineapple is a barbecue superstar.

> **How to do it:** Slice into rings or strips, brush cut sides with a little oil or rum glaze, and grill over medium heat for two to three minutes, until grill-marked.

> **Serving ideas:** Stack alongside pulled pork on a sandwich, dice into salsa for grilled chicken, or eat plain with a sprinkle of cinnamon sugar.

PEACHES

Peaches are quite delicate but shine on the grill.

How to do it: Cut in half and remove pit, brush cut sides with butter or honey, and place cut-side down on the grill for three to five minutes.

Serving ideas: Grilled peaches are great paired with burrata cheese and a drizzle of balsamic; for a quick and delectable dessert, scoop vanilla ice cream over warm peaches.

OTHER FRUITS WORTH GRILLING

Watermelon: Thick slices caramelize beautifully, making a unique topping for a salad.

Apples and pears: This combination makes a great complement to pork chops or works as a sweet side.

Bananas: Soft and caramelized, bananas are practically destined to accompany chocolate.

PRO TIP

- Don't go too far; fruit cooks quickly—and, thus, burns quickly too. A little sear is all you need to up your game.

[68]
INTRODUCTING
DIPS & APPETIZERS

Every pitmaster knows one thing to be true: Guests will get hungry long before the meat is ready. That's where dips and appetizers come into play. Snacks keep guests satisfied without stealing the spotlight from your main attraction. Appetizers also buy you time around the smoker, with the added bonus of ensuring you host like a pro.

TRADITIONAL BBQ APPETIZERS

Spinach and artichoke dip: Creamy and cheesy, this dip is a crowd favorite and very easy to make. Serve warm with grilled bread or chips for delicious dipping.

Buffalo chicken dip: Chicken, cream cheese, hot sauce, and cheddar make this tangy, spicy treat a must for any BBQ. It's addictive!

Pimento cheese spread: This Southern classic can be served on crackers, burgers, or any way you can imagine. Made with cheddar cheese, mayo, and roasted peppers, it's a must.

GRILLED BBQ APPETIZERS

Jalapeño poppers: Halve jalapeños and stuff with cream cheese. For extra flavor, wrap them with bacon and smoke to crisp perfection. A common variation in BBQ circles includes smoked meat, which is referred to by the acronym *ATB*. Despite their somewhat unappetizing name, "Atomic Buffalo Turds" are legendary—and for good reason!

Grilled flatbread with hummus: Brush flatbread with olive oil and throw it on the grill until slightly warm, then serve with your favorite smoky hummus for dipping.

Shrimp skewers: Light and quick to cook up, there's nothing better than shrimp skewers for loosening up appetites.

PRO TIPS

- Keep appetizers small; these are tongue teasers, not entrées.
- Dips are an excellent way to experiment with flavors you plan to use later. For instance, serving a jalapeño chipotle dip before smoked ribs gives guests a hint of what's coming soon.

- Don't forget your vegetarian guests! Providing meat-free appetizers will guarantee everyone feels included, and vegetarian options don't have to be dull. Guacamole, for instance, is universally loved.

[69]
SALADS THAT
AREN'T BORING

At BBQs, salads are often treated as an afterthought; in reality, they're anything but. Great salads cleanse the palate, balance richness, and can even stand alone when given the attention they deserve.

GAME-CHANGING SALADS

Grilled Caesar salad: Cut romaine hearts in half and drizzle with oil, then grill for a splash of color around the edges. Toss the grilled romaine with Caesar dressing, croutons, and parmesan.

Watermelon feta salad: Watermelon cubes tossed with feta, mint, and a drizzle of balsamic glaze make for a refreshing twist.

Southwest salad: Black beans, corn, avocado, tomatoes, and chipotle-lime dressing provide a heftier option with bold flavors.

Pasta salad reimagined: Ditch the heavy mayo for pesto pasta salad with sun-dried tomatoes and arugula.

PRO TIPS

- Balance textures in your salad. Add crunch with nuts or croutons, then combine with creamy ingredients like cheese and avocado for a well-rounded salad.
- Go easy on the dressing. No one wants soggy greens!

- Incorporate grilled elements like corn, peppers, or peaches to maintain the BBQ theme.

[70]
DAZZLING DESSERTS

No BBQ should end without something sweet! Let's be honest: No meal feels complete without dessert, and using the grill, you can bring the BBQ theme straight to the finish line. Desserts are a perfect way to end your BBQ, leaving guests with a sweet memory.

S'MORES: THE CAMPFIRE FAVORITE

Nothing says eating outdoors quite like s'mores! We all know about graham crackers, chocolate, and marshmallows, but creating a BBQ version of s'mores can be even more fun.

> **Peanut butter s'mores:** Spread peanut butter on the graham crackers before assembling the s'more. Wrap in foil and stick on the grill for five minutes.

> **Salted caramel s'mores:** Drizzle caramel sauce over the chocolate for an added level of decadent goodness.

GRILLED BANANAS: SWEET, SMOKY, & SIMPLE

> **Method:** Slice bananas from top to bottom without removing the peels. Stuff with chocolate chips and marshmallows, wrap in foil, and grill for five to seven minutes, until gooey.

> **Serving suggestions:** Serve in bowls and top with crushed nuts or ice cream.

ADDITIONAL GRILL DESSERTS

> **Grilled pound cake:** Grill slices of pound cake and top with fruit or whipped cream.

Campfire apples: Core apples, fill with brown sugar and cinnamon, and wrap in foil before grilling.

PRO TIPS

- Always use indirect heat for desserts. You want them warm, not charred.
- Assemble dessert packets before guests arrive.
- Keep toppings (nuts, sauces, whipped cream) together so that guests can create custom desserts.

CHAPTER EIGHT:
GLOBAL BBQ ADVENTURES

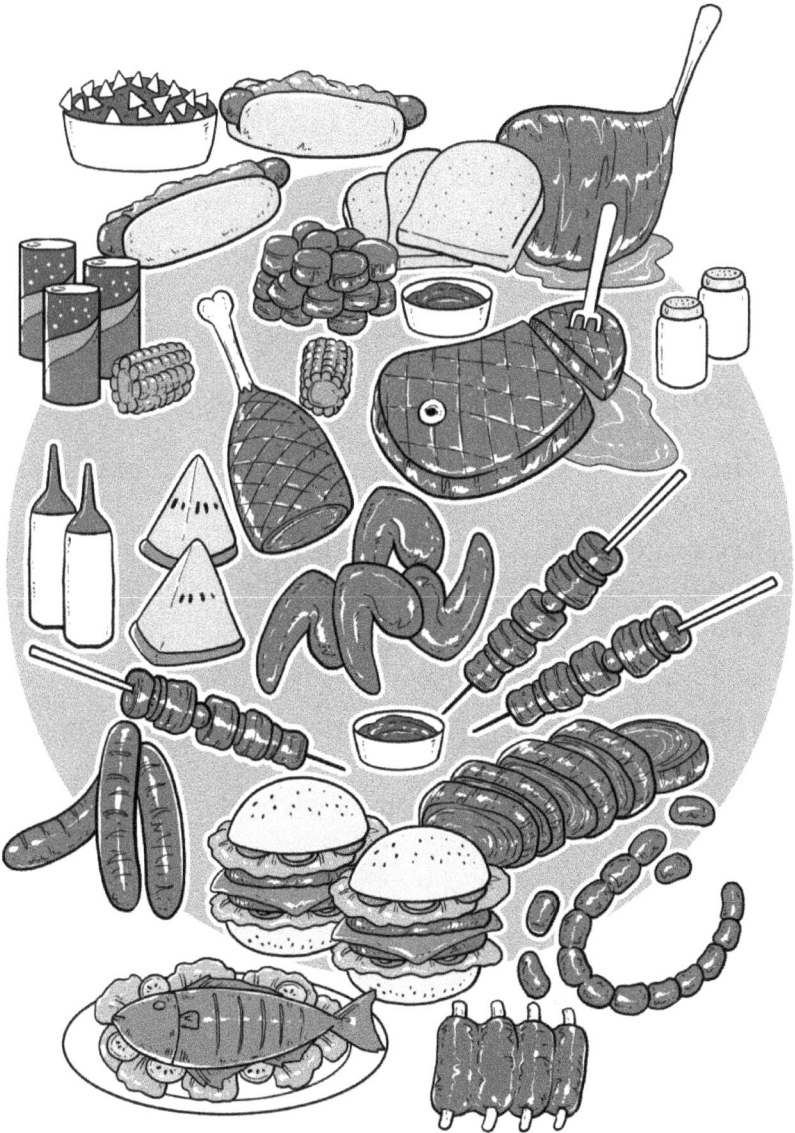

Probably the most exciting aspect of BBQ is its universal nature. Across continents, people have figured out that *fire* plus *meat* equals *happiness*. Every culture has a different approach to BBQ, each with its own unique historical significance, ingredients, and ritual. Diving into these global perspectives doesn't erase classic BBQ by any means—it merely adds to your pitmaster toolbox, giving distinct flair to your brand of entertainment.

[71]
AMERICAN REGIONAL STYLES (TEXAS, MEMPHIS, ETCS.)

In the U.S., BBQ is an identity, a source of pride, and occasionally a rivalry. Each region has its own style, and the more you know about each one, the more versatile a pitmaster you'll be.

TEXAS BBQ

- **Meat:** Beef is king, and brisket is the frontrunner, with ribs a close second.
- **Technique:** Meat is often slow-smoked over oak or mesquite. Seasoning is simple, usually just salt and pepper.
- **Sauce:** Texas BBQ purists believe brisket should stand on its own. When sauce is used, it's thin, tangy, and peppery.

MEMPHIS BBQ

- **Meat:** Pork is the most popular, particularly ribs and pulled pork.
- **Technique:** Aim for slow-smoked over hickory. Ribs are either served "wet" (slathered in sauce) or "dry" (dusted with a spice rub).
- **Sauce:** Sauces are tomato-based, tangy, and subtly sweet.

KANSAS CITY BBQ

- **Meat:** Anything works for Kansas City BBQ, whether ribs, brisket, chicken, or sausage.
- **Technique:** Cook low and slow with heavy hickory smoke.
- **Sauce:** Sauces are thick and sweet, usually with molasses or tomatoes as a base. This is what most Americans envision when they think of BBQ sauce.

CAROLINA BBQ

- **Meat:** Think whole hog or pork shoulder.
- **Technique:** Cook meat slowly over oak or hickory.
- **Sauce:** Sauce is vinegar-based in Eastern North Carolina, but you'll need vinegar-and-tomato "dip" for Lexington-style NC. For mustard-based sauce, head to South Carolina.

[72]
KOREAN BBQ—
BULGOGI BASICS

If the essence of American BBQ is low and slow, Korean BBQ is fast and flavorful. The grill is often front and center of the dining table, where diners take pleasure in cooking their own meat in a communal way. *Bulgogi* literally means "fire meat." Made of thinly sliced beef (generally ribeye or sirloin) marinated in a sweet-savory sauce, bulgogi is cooked quickly over hot coals or flames.

MARINADE BASICS

Marinade is what makes bulgogi special.

- **Soy sauce:** The savory backbone
- **Sugar/honey/pear juice:** Sweeteners that caramelize nicely
- **Garlic and ginger:** Aromatic wonders
- **Sesame oil:** Adds a nutty touch
- **Scallions/sesame seeds:** Fresh finishers

COOKING THE BULGOGI

1. Be sure to marinate beef for at least two hours, overnight if possible.
2. Heat the grill or a cast iron pan until smoking hot.
3. Spread thin slices of beef in a layer, but don't overcrowd.
4. Cook for one to two minutes per side. High heat creates a nice crust while maintaining tenderness.

THE FULL EXPERIENCE

Korean BBQ isn't only about the meat; it's also about the sides, or *banchan*. Think kimchi, pickled daikon, seasoned spinach, and spicy sauce. To get the full experience, wrap your bulgogi in a lettuce leaf with rice, garlic, and chili paste for a fully loaded bite. Korean BBQ brings a playful and engaging attitude to barbecue. It's less about relaxing while waiting for food to cook and more about rolling up your sleeves and cooking together.

PRO TIP

- If you don't have thin-sliced beef, consider cooling the meat to make carving those paper-thin slices easier.

[73]
ARGENTINE ASADO TECHNIQUES

Argentina has created a BBQ culture known as *asado*. More than just a way to prepare food, an asado is a cultural event. The focus is on bringing people together for an extended period of time and having a meal.

Asados are centered around fire or a grill (*parrilla*). A basic parrilla consists of a firebox, fueled by wood or charcoal, and an adjustable grill grate, which slides along a vertical hinge. Argentinians don't dump coal directly under the meat. Instead, they burn wood down to embers in a firebox, then shovel the embers under the grill grate.

Asado is about pacing. An asado starts with sausages and offal, while big cuts take time to cook. Generally, plenty of wine is consumed while guests exchange conversation and laughter before the main meat is served.

- **Beef:** Argentina is a cattle country, and its beef is second to none. Look for ribs, short ribs, flank, and sirloin.
- **Chorizo and morcilla:** Sausage and blood sausage are also common.
- **Offal (achuras):** Sweetbreads, kidney, and intestines are often included.

THE COOKING METHOD

- Slow grill at low and constant heat.
- Use very little seasoning other than coarse salt. The meat and smoke speak for themselves.
- Meat is cooked whole, then sliced at the table and shared among everyone.

CHIMICHURRI: THE ESSENTIAL SAUCE

Every Argentine asado features chimichurri, a bright and herbaceous sauce. The classic version includes parsley, garlic, oregano, olive oil, vinegar, and chili flakes. It's bright, it's fresh, and it perfectly balances the rich flavor of beef.

PRO TIP

- Don't flip constantly. Argentine grillers slow-cook meat for a long time during asados, but only flip once. Waiting brings tenderness.

[74]
BRAZILIAN-CHURRASCO SKEWERS

BBQ in Brazil isn't a meal; it's a performance. *Churrasco* (Portuguese for "barbecue") is a centuries-old cooking method from the gaucho (cowboy) culture of southern Brazil. Over the years, churrasco has evolved into a treasured form of contemporary culinary art recognized in Brazilian steakhouses across the globe.

Traditionally, churrasco is cooked over an open flame on a long, open grilling surface. Modern versions feature a rotisserie-style skewer revolving slowly over a bed of charcoal. Each cut of meat is seasoned, placed on large skewers, and rotisserie grilled over intense flame. Skewers are up to four feet long, perfect for large cuts of meat.

THE MEATS

Brazilian churrasco is all about variety.

- **Picanha:** The star cut is beef top sirloin cap with the fat cap still intact, seasoned only with coarse salt and grilled to medium rare.
- **Other cuts:** Look for sausages (linguiça), chicken hearts, lamb, pork ribs, and sirloin.
- **Vegetarian options:** Peppers, onions, and cheese (queijo coalho) are also placed on skewers to be grilled.

THE EXPERIENCE

In Brazilian steakhouses (churrascarias), servers roam the dining room with skewers and slice meat directly onto diners' plates. At home, churrasco is a social event; friends gather around the churrasqueira, eating in waves as each meat finishes cooking.

PRO TIP

- Don't over-season your churrasco. Trust the meat, fire, and fat. A couple of cracks of salt and a proper sear beat complicated marinades.

[75]
SOUTH AFRICAN
BRAAI TRADITIONS

If BBQ is a meal in America, then in South Africa, it's a way of life. The *braai* (Afrikaans for "grill") is so culturally important that it has an annual public holiday on September 24: National Braai Day. Braai is a proud embodiment of togetherness, conversation, and South African identity.

While many BBQ traditions allow for gas grilling, braai purists only accept wood or charcoal. Hardwood is the fuel of choice. Rooikrans and kameeldoring are popular for their heavy smoke and long burn. Since fire is the most important aspect, cooking with gas isn't usually considered a true braai.

Braai is as much about the gathering as it is about food. The braai master tends the fire with pride as everyone else relaxes with drinks, chatting, as the food cooks. Fire is part of the entertainment, and people stick around the flames long after the food has finished cooking.

THE DIFFERENT MEATS

- **Boerewors:** Coiled sausage made from beef, pork, and spices is juicy, flavorful, and a must-have for the braai.
- **Steaks and lamb chops:** These are usually prepared simply with salt, pepper, or a local spice blend.
- **Chicken and fish:** As occasional accompaniments, chicken and fish may be marinated in peri-peri sauce for added kick.

- **Sosaties:** Meat, usually lamb or chicken, is marinated in curry, then threaded onto a skewer. Often, chunks of dried fruit are added (usually apricots).

THE SIDE DISHES

Braai isn't just for meat. Popular side dishes include:

- **Pap:** A maize porridge that resembles grits, usually served with tomato sauce
- **Chakalaka:** A spicy bean-and-vegetable relish
- **Salads:** Potato, bean, or beetroot

PRO TIP

- Respect the fire. A braai is an art form requiring each generation to hand down the skill of controlling the coals. Part of the journey to becoming a braai master is judging the moment when the fire is ready.

[76]
JAMAICAN JERK CHICKEN

Few BBQ plates have as much personality as Jamaican jerk chicken. Smoky, spicy, aromatic, and unapologetically flavorful, jerk is undoubtedly one of the Caribbean's most recognizable culinary exports.

Jerk cooking goes back to the Maroons, enslaved Africans who escaped to the mountains of Jamaica. They figured out how to preserve, then season meats with local spices before cooking them over pimento wood (allspice) for heat and flavor. This process, developed as a matter of survival, eventually evolved into a powerful food culture.

THE MARINADE

Jerk chicken shines because of its marinade paste:

- **Scotch bonnet peppers:** Fiery heat with fruity undertones
- **Allspice:** Responsible for the warm, peppery flavor representative of jerk
- **Thyme:** Provides earthiness and balance.
- **Garlic, ginger, and scallions:** The fragrant backbone
- **Soy sauce and lime:** Savory and sour

THE COOKING METHOD

Meat is typically marinated for a few hours or overnight to allow for flavor development. Plus, jerk isn't just grilled but also smoked as well. Meat is placed on green pimento wood racks above smoldering coals. Pimento wood gives jerk its signature smell, and indirect heat results in juicy, evenly cooked meat. While pimento wood can be hard to come by, a variety of additives—allspice berries, bay leaves, and hickory or applewood—can still get you that authentic jerk flavor.

THE FLAVOR

Jerk chicken layers smoky and spicy flavors to make each bite sweet, sour, fruity, savory, and herbal at the same time. It is BBQ that demands your attention. Jerk chicken is commonly served with:

- **Rice and peas:** Coconut rice with red kidney beans
- **Fried plantains:** Sweet and caramelized to counterbalance heat
- **Festival:** Fried cornmeal dumplings, slightly sweet and great for soaking up sauce

PRO TIP

- Keep it hot—Scotch bonnets are the real deal. To keep jerk chicken from burning the faces off your guests, you can balance the heat with brown sugar or honey.

[77]
INDIAN TANDOORI
ON THE GRILL

When you think of Indian food, curry or naan may come to mind first, but one of Indian cuisine's best contributions to the world of grilling is tandoori cooking. Traditionally, this is done in a tandoor, a cylindrical clay oven fueled by charcoal that creates high, dry heat. The oven cooks the outside of the meat quickly and seals in the juiciness. However, it's possible to achieve tandoori on your backyard grill without a clay oven.

THE MARINADE

Tandoori uses flavorful marinades. Chicken is the most common meat used, usually scored so that the marinade can penetrate the meat. You can also use lamb, paneer (cheese), or even fish.

- **Base:** Yogurt enzymes to tenderize meat and add creaminess
- **Spices:** Garam masala, cumin, coriander, turmeric, paprika, and chili powder
- **Aromatics:** Garlic, ginger, and lemon juice
- **Signature color:** Traditionally from red chiles, paprika, and turmeric

PRO TIP

On a grill set up for two-zone cooking, sear the chicken over direct high heat, then move to indirect heat to cook it through. Don't fear the char—those blackened bits are full of flavor!

Don't skimp on marinating time! The best depth of flavor is achieved by marinating overnight. The cooling raita (yogurt sauce) and naan balance the spice.

[78]
AUSTRALIAN
BARBIE TIPS

In Australia, BBQ truly is an institution, and "barbie" is synonymous with a gathering, whether at the beach, a park, or at home. While similarities exist between Australian barbecue and how BBQ is understood in America, there are notable differences as well.

In terms of culture, Aussie BBQ is casual. Friends bring drinks, cooking is done in rings, and everything is shared. Aussie BBQ is less about low-and-slow smoking and more about a quick, convenient, and tasty meal enjoyed with a few drinks and mates.

THE SETUP

- **Gas grills:** Gas is primarily for convenience, but Australians also have a cult following for charcoal.
- **Flat plates (hotplates):** These are perfect for on-site cooking of eggs, onions, or seafood.

THE MEATS

- **Sausages (snags):** Basic pork or beef sausages, served on white bread with onion and tomato sauce (ketchup), are iconic in Australian barbecues.
- **Lamb chops:** Australia is one of the largest producers of lamb, making it a staple at the barbie.
- **Seafood:** Shrimp, fish fillets, and scallops
- **Steaks and burgers:** Always present, cooked quickly

[79]
MEXICAN
CARNE ASADA

Very few foods exemplify social grilling like Mexican carne asada, which literally means "grilled meat." Most commonly using beef (usually skirt or flank), carne asada is marinated, grilled over high heat, and sliced thinly. The meat is meant to be enjoyed in a taco or burrito, but you can also eat it just with salsa and tortilla chips.

THE MARINADE

Carne asada is bold but balanced:

- **Acid:** Lime or orange juice to tenderize
- **Savory:** Garlic, onion, soy sauce, or Worcestershire
- **Herbs and spices:** Cilantro, cumin, chili powder
- **Heat:** Fresh or dried chilies

Marinating also infuses flavor and keeps the beef from drying out, since skirt steak is a lean cut.

THE COOKING

1. Grill over direct high heat. Carne asada is about char and caramelization, not low-and-slow smoking.
2. Cook to medium or medium rare. Overcooking skirt steak can make it tough.
3. Always cut against the grain for tenderness.

THE FEAST

Carne asada is usually served with:

- Fresh tortillas (corn or flour)
- Guacamole, salsa, or pico de gallo
- Rice and beans
- Grilled scallions, peppers, or nopales (cactus)

PRO TIP

- Be sure to rest before slicing; just a few minutes will make the meat juicier and easier to cut.

[80]
FUSION IDEAS &
MIXING CULTURES

The experimental characteristics of contemporary BBQ are among its many pleasures. You don't have to be constrained by any particular tradition. Fusion is an opportunity to experiment across cultures and traditions, allowing you to be both pitmaster and mad scientist.

EXAMPLES OF FUSION BBQ

- **Korean-Mexican tacos:** Bulgogi beef wrapped in tortillas with kimchi salsa (a staple food-truck success in Los Angeles that took off worldwide).
- **Tandoori wings:** Chicken wings dipped in tandoori spices and smoked low and slow, southern style.
- **Jerk pork belly burnt ends:** Traditional Jamaican jerk marinade with Kansas City burnt ends: sweet, smoky, spicy, and really tasty.
- **Chimichurri burgers:** American burgers topped with traditional Argentine chimichurri sauce, where bright herbs add a sharp contrast to the richness of beef
- **BBQ ramen:** Grilled pork belly or brisket with Japanese ramen broth to add smoky flavor.

PRO TIPS

- Understand and respect each tradition first before fusing it with another.
- Don't overload with competing flavors. Choose one culture or tradition to dominate and another as support.

- Tacos, burgers, skewers, or sandwiches are good engines for fusion.
- Fusion isn't about being gimmicky; it's about respecting global flavors while creating something new.

CHAPTER NINE:
PITFALLS & PRO TIPS

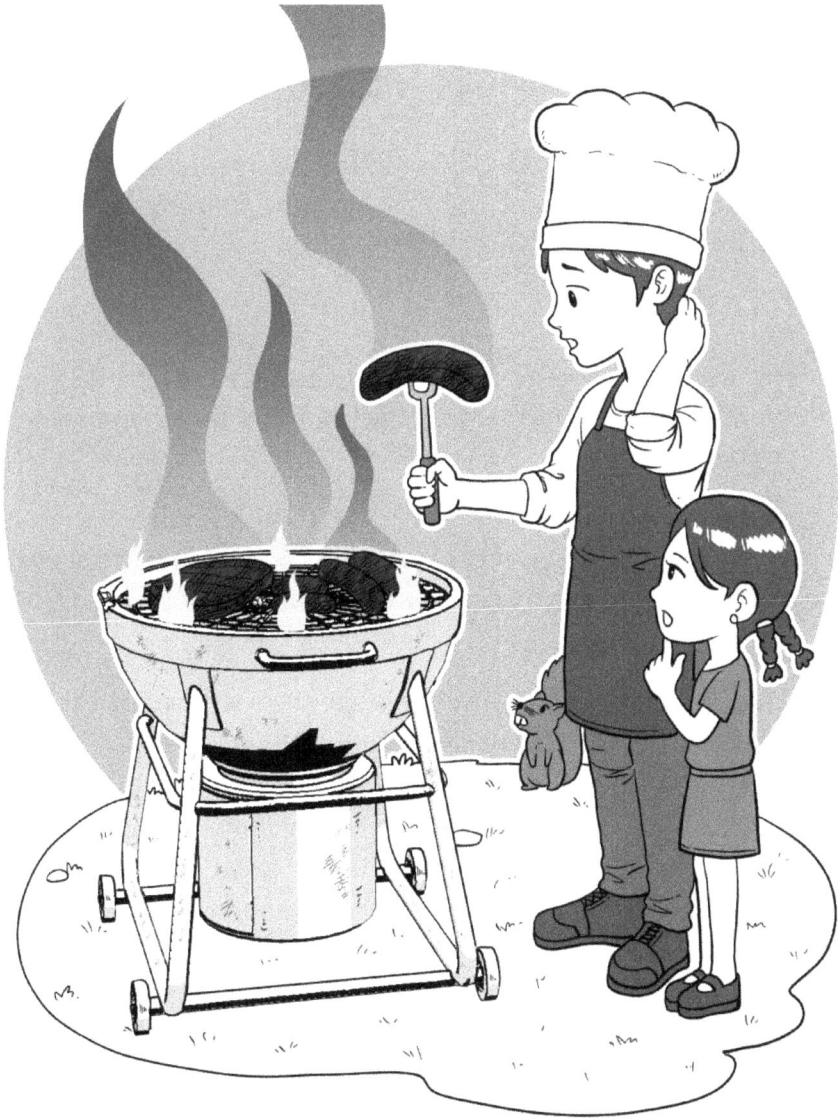

Regardless of your skill level at the grill, things can go wrong. You can burn a slab of meat, a storm can blow in, or grease can build up. Suddenly, your BBQ confidence takes a hit. The good news is that most BBQ disasters can be avoided with the right knowledge. This chapter discusses common mistakes, weatherproofing, and maintenance tips needed to enjoy BBQ in any season.

[81]
COMMON MISTAKES

Even the most experienced pitmasters make mistakes. The key is understanding the source of the problem and fixing it before your guests end up chewing shoe leather.

FLARE-UPS

Flare-ups are caused by grease drips hitting flames. While a little flare-up can add some smokiness, too much will turn your steak into charcoal.

> **Fix:** Create a "safe zone" on the grill with no direct flame so that you can move meat quickly if your blaze gets out of control. Trim excess fat from each cut before putting it on the grill.

> **Don't use water:** Spraying water on a flare-up spreads grease and ash, which can actually make it worse. Instead, close the lid to extinguish the flame.

OVERCOOKING

Nothing ruins a great cut of meat faster than drying it out.

> **Fix:** Use a meat thermometer to take the guesswork out of temperatures and know your temperatures. Pull meat off the grill slightly below it reaches your target temperature; carryover cooking will raise internal temperature by a few degrees while resting.

Pro hack: For chicken breasts and lean pork, brining will keep the meat juicy, making it more forgiving of mistakes.

UNDER-SEASONING

You can cook the meat perfectly, but if it's bland, it's a wasted opportunity.

Fix: Don't be timid about seasoning! Season early, season generously. (See Chapter 4 for tips on adding flavor.)

[82]
WEATHERPROOFING YOUR BBQ

Rain, wind, and cold don't have to cancel your cookout. With proper setup, you can grill year-round, come hell or high water.

GRILLING IN RAIN

Lid on: Rain cools the grill surface, so preheat longer and keep the lid closed as much as possible to keep from lowering the heat.

Shelter: Use a grill canopy, umbrella, awning, or place under a roof overhang, but never grill indoors. Carbon monoxide is deadly!

Fuel tip: Bring extra coals or wood, as wet conditions put a damper on burning time.

COLD-WEATHER GRILLING

Preheat longer: Cold air robs heat (shocking, we know), so give your grill more time to reach the desired temperature.

Fuel efficiency: Pick simple, familiar recipes that cook up quickly, and expect to use more fuel. Gas grills often struggle with fuel efficiency in subzero temperatures, whereas charcoal retains heat better in the cold. If you do use propane, make sure to replace any leaky hoses ahead of time.

Dress the part: Bundle up! Insulating gloves that allow dexterity keep you both safe and comfortable.

WINDY CONDITIONS

Wind blockers: Put your grill against a wall or use a windscreen. Position your grill so that the flame faces away from the wind.

Charcoal: Wind can cause charcoal to burn hotter and faster, so vent accordingly.

Gas: Always light a gas grill with the lid open. If the wind blows out the flame, close the valves quickly to avoid gas buildup. Wait for the smell of gas to dissipate before relighting; otherwise, you may lose your eyebrows — or worse.

Pro Tip

Invest in an all-weather grill cover to protect your grill from rust, rain, and UV rays. A quality cover will last for years. Less-than-ideal weather doesn't have to mean that grilling cannot continue. True pitmasters know that, rain or shine, the show must go on.

[83]
CLEANING & MAINTENANCE ROUTINES

A dirty grill isn't only disgusting. It also affects flavor, increases the risk of flare-ups, and shortens the life of your equipment. Just as you perform regular maintenance on your car, you should also maintain your grill.

AFTER EACH COOK

Brush the grates: Scrub grates with a quality brush while the grill is still hot; again, avoid old wire-bristle brushes that shed harmful metal pieces. Bristle-free brushes, coil brushes, scrapers, and grill stones are all good options.

Oil the grates: After cleaning, oil the grill grates lightly to prevent rusting and make your next cook easier.

WEEKLY/MONTHLY CARE

Dump the ash catcher: Regularly clear ashes from charcoal grills, as ash holds moisture and, thus, can cause metal to corrode.

Deep clean/scrub: For gas grills, remove the burner cover and tray and soak them in warm soapy water. For charcoal, remove the grates and clean the inside with a scraper or putty knife.

Check the gas lines: If you have a propane grill, regularly check for leaks by brushing soapy water on hoses and connections, then slowly opening the valve. If you see bubbles forming, you have a leak.

MAINTENANCE BY SEASON

Reseason cast iron: If you use cast iron grates, reseason them by applying a thin layer of oil, just like you would a skillet.

Rust hunt: Sand off any rust spots, and apply high-temperature grill paint if spots persist.

Hardware inspection: Tighten screws, check hinges, and ensure wheels/legs are stable.

Pro Tip

If there is stubborn grime on your grill, run it on high for fifteen minutes, then scrub. Heat separates debris, making clean-up much easier. You can also cut an onion in half and rub it on hot grates; the onion's acidity lifts charred bits and leaves a subtle flavor.

Cleaning your grill is not only a matter of BBQ hygiene — it's also about performance and safety. Food will taste better, fires will burn consistently, and your investment will last longer. Flare-ups, rainstorms, and rust won't stand a chance when you use these hacks.

[84]
FOOD SAFETY

No matter how delicious your BBQ looks, if everyone ends up sick, you're done. When you're working with raw meat and fire, food safety is not an option — it's mandatory.

The USDA has defined the "danger zone" as temperatures between 40°F and 140°F. This is where bacteria flourish. Always keep raw foods cold until you're ready to prepare, and don't let cooked food sit outdoors for more than an hour or two. Food safety may not be glamorous, but it's what separates amateur grillers from professional pitmasters.

SAFE COOKING TEMPERATURES

- Poultry (all cuts, including ground): 165°F
- Ground beef, pork, lamb, veal: 160°F
- Steaks, chops, roasts (beef, lamb, pork): 145°F with a three-minute rest
- Fish: 145°F

A good meat thermometer is a pitmaster's best friend, but don't just poke around aimlessly. Insert it in the thickest part of the product without touching the bone.

PRO TIPS

- **Separate items:** Don't use the same cutting board or knife for both meat and veggies.
- **Dedicated utensils:** Avoid touching cooked food with the same tongs you used for raw meat.
- **Wash your hands:** Wash your hands thoroughly with soap and warm water each and every time you switch tasks.
- **Marinades:** Don't reuse marinades without boiling them first.

[85]
FIXING DRY MEAT
AFTER THE FACT

The last thing any pitmaster wants to do is pull that savory steak off the grill only to find it dry as the desert or discover that their beautiful brisket is chewy and parched because it rested too long. Never fear — with some tricks of the trade, you can rescue dry meat from the brink of disaster.

The important thing to remember is that pros mess up too. Sometimes, you won't be able to fully fix a dry disaster, but you can disguise it for sure. Chop it up for use in chili, stew, or fried rice. Dry brisket, for instance, makes great hash. Never throw away meat.

QUICK FIXES

Broth bath: Slice meat and put it on low heat in warm beef or chicken broth to restore moisture and flavor.

Butter baste: Melt butter and herbs (rosemary, thyme, garlic), then drizzle over slices. Fat does a good job of masking dryness.

BBQ sauce rescue: Chop up the meat, mix it with sauce, and serve in sliders or tacos. No one can resist a saucy pulled pork sandwich!

PREEMPTIVE HACKS

- **Rest meat properly:** Always let meat rest after grilling to allow juices to redistribute, preventing dry cuts.
- **Brine or marinade:** For lean meats like chicken breast or pork chops, brining ahead of time will help keep moisture inside the meat.
- **Low and slow:** Things like brisket and pork shoulder need low-and-slow cooking to break down collagen.

PRO TIP

Always keep a pan of broth or stock on your grill setup. If something is looking dry mid-cook, give it a splash or spritz to keep moisture levels up.

[86]
ECO-FRIENDSLY
BBQ PRACTICES

Barbeque is about fire, meat, and fun, not trashing the planet. With some smart decisions, you can lessen waste and lower emissions, all while throwing a great cookout. Eco-friendly BBQ isn't sacrificing flavor; it's grilling mindfully. Fire tastes better when you know you aren't harming the future of the next generation you help feed.

With these hacks, your BBQing reputation is covered, from food safety and rescuing dry meat to sustainability and common-sense practices. A true pitmaster knows how to BBQ—but more importantly, he knows how to protect the health of his guests, get the most out of every ingredient, and respect the environment.

Ultimately, BBQ isn't only about feeding humans today; it's also about securing the ability to feed others for years to come.

FUEL OPTIONS

Charcoal: Lump charcoal burns cleaner than briquettes, which contain binders (starch, sawdust, etc.) and additives.

Sustainable wood: Check for FSC-certified hardwoods, or use local wood instead of imported.

Propane: Gas produces fewer emissions than charcoal, but some may argue that the trade-off is taste.

Pellets: We all know that recycling is good for the planet, and pellets are generally created from leftover sawdust—so they're efficient and eco-friendly!

CUT WASTE

Reusable: Avoid paper plates and plastic forks. Buy some durable outdoor dishware.

Recycle and compost: Beer cans are easy to recycle, while food scraps can be composted.

Portion control: To avoid food waste, only cook as much as you need. Leftovers are great, but don't grill too much and throw food away.

ECO-FRIENDLY MEAT

Buy from a local butcher or farm that practices sustainable animal husbandry. It's a win-win: You reduce transport distance, receive fresh meat, and support your local community.

Also, consider incorporating more veggies or plant-based proteins. Grilled zucchini, mushrooms, or jackfruit can be just as noteworthy as ribs and brisket.

WATER & CLEANING

- Don't wash your grill with a hose every time. Scrape, wipe down, and spot-clean instead of wasting gallons of water.
- Natural cleaners like vinegar and baking soda work just as well or better than dangerous chemicals.

PRO TIP

Use residual heat from the grill to burn off residue after cooking, then shut it down. That way, you conserve fuel and reduce waste in one go.

[87]
BUDGET BBQ FOR
BROKE WEEKENDS

Eating like a king doesn't have to empty your wallet. Some of the best BBQ comes from affordable cuts and creative, inexpensive side dishes. BBQ has always been about maximizing what you have. A pitmaster's magic is taking simple ingredients and creating amazing meals.

AFFORDABLE CUTS & SEASONING

- **Chicken thighs and drumsticks:** Good value, delicious, and very forgiving
- **Pork shoulder:** The perfect cut for pulled pork that can feed a crowd on a budget
- **Skirt/flank steak:** Less expensive than ribeye and provides huge flavor if marinated properly
- **Sausages:** Classic, inexpensive, and it's easy to mix it up with variety packs
- **Rubs:** Homemade rubs cost cents on the dollar compared to store-bought. All you need is salt, sugar, paprika, and garlic powder, which you likely have in your pantry already.

- **Seasonal vegetables:** Use seasonal vegetables and fruits for side dishes. Grilled zucchini, corn, or peppers fill out a meal, and they're especially affordable when in season.

PRO TIPS

Plan meals around leftovers. Pork shoulder may be pricey on the front end, but when used in sandwiches, tacos, and fried rice over the week, it's more cost effective than fast food.

[88]
ENTERTAINING
LARGE GROUPS

Grilling for a few friends is easy. Grilling for thirty, however, is a whole other ballgame, and this is where planning and strategy come into play.

PLAN YOUR MENU

1. Choose one or two "star" meats (ribs, brisket, etc.) and two or three sides.
2. Add a filler protein (sausages or burgers, preferably). Cheap, fast-cooking, and easy to serve, they keep people satisfied while you finish up larger cuts of meat.

SCALE YOUR SETUP

- Use multiple heat zones: one side for high-heat grilling, the other for low-and-slow smoking.
- Prepare warming trays, or keep finished meats in a cooler insulated with foil and towels.

KEEP GUESTS BUSY

Hungry, impatient guests can stress you out when they hover as you manage multiple food items at once. Providing appetizers (like we discussed in Chapter 7) can buy you time, and when you add drinks and music to the mix, guests will have plenty to occupy their attention.

PRO TIP

Delegate. Ask a friend to manage drinks, another to plate and serve sides, allowing you to focus on the meat. A pitmaster isn't just a cook, after all — they're the conductor of a backyard orchestra.

[89]
HANGOVER CURES
WITH LEFTOVER BBQ

Occasionally, a night of beer, smoke, and laughter can lead to a rough morning. The good news is that BBQ is the gift that keeps on giving, and leftovers can make for the best hangover cures.

BBQ BREAKFAST IDEAS

- **Brisket and eggs:** Cut leftover brisket into hash with potatoes, onions, and fried eggs.
- **Pulled pork omelet:** Mix shredded pork with cheese and jalapeños in fluffy eggs.
- **BBQ breakfast sandwich:** Add all the sausage, egg, and cheese you desire, along with BBQ sauce, on a toasted bun.

COMFORT FOOD POSSIBILITIES

- **BBQ ramen:** Take instant noodles, shred chicken or pork into the broth, and add splashes of chili oil and lime.
- **Grease bomb tacos:** Shred leftover steak and add eggs, hot sauce, and cheese inside some tortillas.
- **Grilled cheese with BBQ:** Put pulled pork or brisket on sliced bread, add cheese, then push together and slap in a skillet for a melty, salty meal.

PRO TIP

Hydration is the best cure for post-BBQ woes. Pair these meals with fruit juice, coconut water, or – if you're feeling adventurous – a bloody mary.

[90]
UPGRADING
SKILLS

Once you've mastered your backyard grill, you might be curious to explore beyond it. That's where competitions and BBQ classes can steer you.

COMPETITIONS

Local BBQ contests: Start small. A little friendly competition will put your skills to the test while introducing you to a community of fellow pitmasters.

Sanctioned events: Organizations like the Kansas City Barbeque Society hold serious competitions with strict rules and judging criteria. Contestants are judged on the "holy four": brisket, ribs, chicken, and pork shoulder.

What you'll learn: When it comes to BBQ competitions, timing, presentation, and consistency are just as important as taste. Competing will tighten your discipline and up your game.

BBQ CLASSES

In person: Many pitmasters do weekend workshops that teach everything from rubs and smoking to advanced techniques.

Online: Online classes are an inexpensive and flexible way to learn directly from experienced pitmasters who provide hacks, tricks, and techniques. This option is perfect if you live in a remote area and can't travel.

What you'll gain: In addition to tasty recipes, you'll learn about fire control, flavor theory, and troubleshooting under high pressure.

Pro Tip

Even if you never compete, learning about competitive BBQ will take your backyard game to higher levels of precision, confidence, and swagger. Competitions and classes remind us that BBQ is both an art and a science. Pitmasters never stop learning, and that's what makes the journey so addictive.

CHAPTER TEN:
PAIRINGS & PARTIES

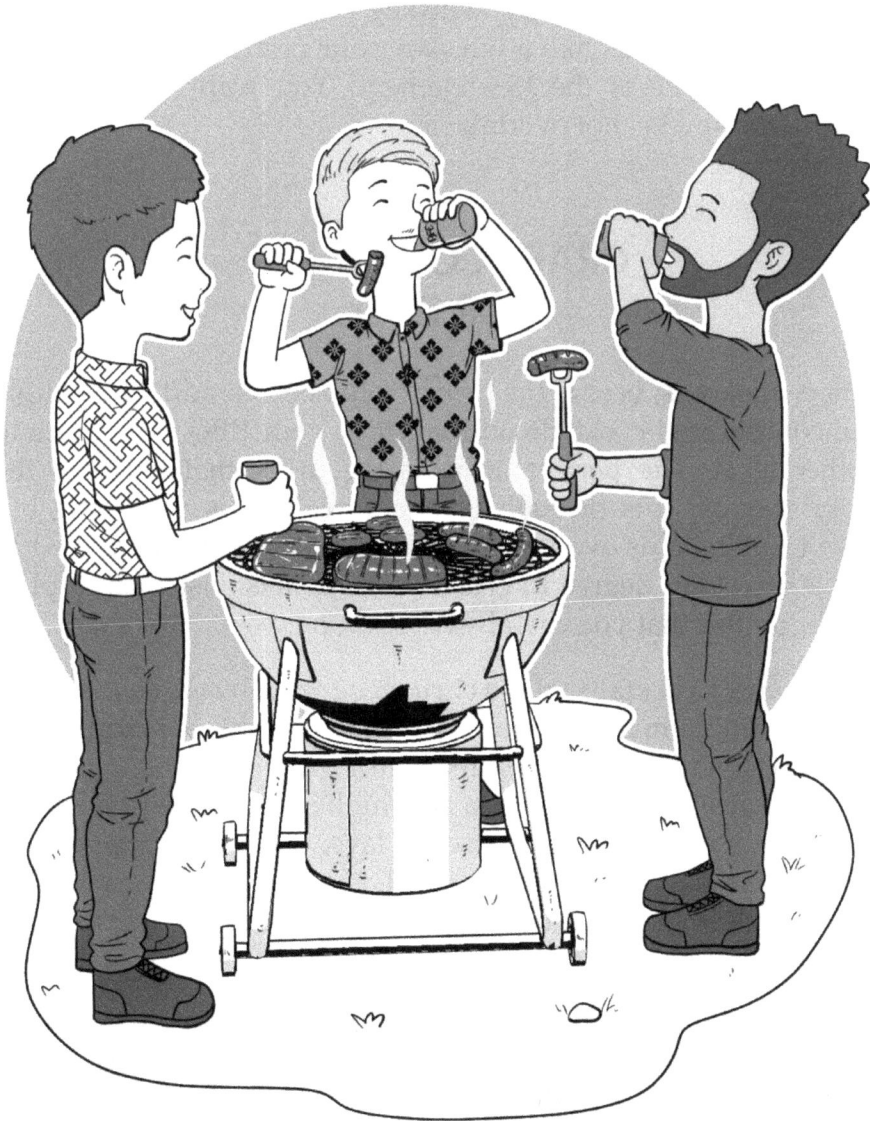

When it comes to BBQ, what you have in your glass is just as important as what's on the grill. The right drink does far more than wash down the food; it elevates the overall BBQ experience. Whether you're a beer guy, a whiskey sipper, or you're looking for some great non-alcoholic options, you can find a great pairing for every BBQ.

There's no need to get fancy; whiskey is great neat, on the rocks, and even in cocktails like a whiskey sour or old-fashioned. Most critically, balance is the key element. You want the drink to enhance the smoke, not overtake it.

[91]
CRAFT COCKTAILS
FOR BBQ

In most cookouts, beer is the drink of choice, but adding a couple of uncomplicated cocktails will improve your BBQ experience to another level. The perfect drink is the drink that balances the smoky flavors, cuts through the richness, and is refreshing but doesn't outshine or overwhelm the food. And you don't need to have a mixology degree to create some drinks, just a handful of classic combos that you can always rely on.

To get started, cocktails with a citrus base will always be a winner; consider simple margaritas or mojitos, two upper tier drinks that bring brightness and are perfect with grilled meats. A smoky mezcal mule is also a great idea as it highlights all the rich flavors of the pit, yet the ginger adds an extra layer of depth. Alternatively, if you want something sweeter and you don't mind exercising your southern charm, a bourbon lemonade or a spiked iced tea would be a great idea to couple with sticky pulled pork or ribs.

Don't forget about your non-drinker guests; mocktail drinks made with fresh fruit, herbs, and soda water are a fun way to make sure everyone is included. In the end, cocktails are meant to be fun and flavor-driven decisions, not complicated and fancy crafting methods. Keep focusing on freshness, keep it simple, and make the drink another fun and exciting spark at your next BBQ.

[92]
WHISKEY & BBQ
HARMONY

If beer is the casual cousin of BBQ, then whiskey is the sophisticated uncle. There's nothing quite like sipping whiskey between bites of smoky meat for pure intensity and depth. There's no need to get fancy; whiskey is great neat, on the rocks, and even in cocktails like a whiskey sour or old-fashioned. Most critically, balance is the key element. You want the drink to enhance the smoke, not overtake it.

PAIRING BY STYLE

- **Bourbon:** The sweet vanilla-and-caramel characteristics of bourbon match well with ribs or pulled pork, and the char from oak barrels can be reminiscent of BBQ smoke.
- **Rye whiskey:** Spicy and sharp, rye matches beautifully with brisket and other beef cuts.
- **Peated scotch:** The complex, smoky, and earthy flavors in peated scotch complement rich game meat such as venison and lamb.
- **Irish whiskey:** Smooth and light, Irish whiskey is the perfect complement to chicken and seafood.

PRO TIP

Cooking with whiskey is a great way to up your game! Whiskey-glazed ribs or a bourbon-infused BBQ sauce will gain your cookout legendary status.

[93]
NON-ALCOHOLIC OPTIONS
THAT DON'T SUCK

Plenty of people don't drink alcohol, and even beer-lovers may occasionally want something refreshing and alcohol free. Fortunately, non-alcoholic drinks can be anything but boring.

FUN & REFRESHING OPTIONS

- **Sparkling citrus water:** Customize with lemon, lime, or grapefruit slices.
- **Homemade lemonade or limeade:** Freshly squeezed, slightly tart goodness goes well with smoky meats.
- **Iced tea:** Iced tea is a classic southern beverage, sweet or no. Mint or peach can add some flair.
- **Mocktails:** Virgin mojitos (mint and lime) are extremely refreshing, and "smoked" mocktails using herbs and fruit can feel as sophisticated as alcoholic options.
- **Non-alcoholic beer or cider:** Many craft breweries produce high-end versions of alcohol-free beverages that closely resemble their alcoholic counterparts.

PRO TIP

Serve non-alcoholic beverages in the same way as alcoholic beverages: frosted mugs, fancy glassware, and garnishes. Presentation makes every guest feel included.

[94]
TAILGATING BBQ
SETUPS

Few things shout BBQ culture louder than a tailgate party. Whether it's before a football game or a concert, hanging out in a parking lot while you fire up a grill is a ritual unto itself.

WHAT YOU'LL NEED

- **Portable grill:** Charcoal for taste or gas for convenience
- **Cooler:** A place to store meat, drinks, and sides until you're ready to go
- **Mobile Furniture:** Chairs and tables for food prep and comfort
- **Shade:** Pop-up canopies or umbrellas for enjoying the sun

MENU IDEAS

Don't overthink it. Tailgate food should be easy, portable, and crowd-friendly. Think burgers, sausages, wings, skewers, and foil-packet sides. Nobody wants to wait two hours for brisket before kickoff.

PRO TIP

Prep as much as you can at home. Marinate meat, chop veggies, and stow everything in zipper bags. This way, you'll spend considerably less time fumbling around in a hot parking lot, leaving you time to soak up the vibe.

[95]
BACKYARD PARTY PLANNING

Your yard is your territory, and nothing says "pitmaster" quite like putting on a backyard BBQ that everyone talks about. However, even when you're on your home turf, any good party requires careful planning.

SET THE SCENE

> **Seating and lighting:** Make sure you have enough chairs, tables, and adequate lighting for when the sun goes down. String lights are a perfect way to set the mood quickly.

Music: Have a good sound system and prepare a playlist for background and energy.

Kid zone: If you're throwing a kid-friendly bash, provide lawn games or bubbles to keep them engaged.

FOOD FLOW

- Pick one or two meat centerpieces (brisket, ribs) and compensate with quicker grilling items (burgers, wings, kabobs).
- Prep sides ahead of time: coleslaw, potato salad, grilled corn.
- Set up a clean, fully stocked drink station for your guests to grab their own beverages.

PRO TIP

Cook more food than you think you'll need. Leftovers are no problem, but running out of food is.

[96]
GIFT IDEAS FOR
BBQ BROS

BBQ is a fraternity. Whether it's for a birthday, Father's Day, or another holiday, you can't go wrong with BBQ-themed gifts. In addition to showing you care, BBQ gifts are a great way to provide a present that won't just sit on a shelf. More than simple tools, they're an investment in the lifestyle.

AFFORDABLE BUT THOUGHTFUL

- **Quality tongs or spatula:** Tools a pitmaster can't ever have enough of
- **Personalized apron or cutting board:** Adds flair and sense of ownership

- **Wood chips or pellets:** Helps the recipient discover an entirely new smoke experience

MID-RANGE GEAR

- **Digital meat thermometer:** Essential to precision
- **Cast iron skillet or griddle:** Allows for grilling versatility
- **Barbecue rub or sauce sampler pack:** A set of flavorful gifts to inspire creativity

BIG TICKET ITEMS

- **Smoker or pellet grill upgrade:** A gift that will get legendary recognition
- **Vouchers for BBQ classes:** A chance to take their cooking to the next level
- **Custom knife:** Nothing's better than a razor-sharp carving blade

PRO TIP

You can never go wrong with a six-pack of craft beer or a bottle of bourbon to send along.

[97]
BUILDING A
HOME BBQ PIT

Every grill master wants a permanent monument to fire and smoke, but it doesn't have to be some elaborate edifice. A backyard pit can be as simple as a stack of cinder blocks or as robust as a brick-lined smoker with a chimney. Build your pit near a seating area, but not too close to the house. Safety, airflow, and a place to gather are important considerations.

- **Basic build:** Stack cinder blocks into a *U* shape, put a metal grate on top, and you're in business.

- **Permanent construction:** A brick or stone pit will last a generation and easily double as an outdoor fireplace.

[98]
SEASONAL BBQ & WINTER GRILLING

Snow cover shouldn't be a reason for your grill to hibernate. Winter grilling is a little more difficult, but well worth it. There's something primal about tending fire in the cold, the steam rising off sizzling meat, against the frosty backdrop. Winter BBQ isn't just cooking; it's bragging rights.

- **Keep the lid closed:** Cold air brings down grill temps quickly, so the less you lift the lid, the better.
- **Fuel:** You'll burn more fuel in winter, so plan for it.
- **Dress for the occasion:** Gloves, boots, and a warm coat are a must so that you can focus on food.

[99]
HEALTHY TWEAKS

BBQ may be a stereotypically indulgent meal, but with a few small tweaks, BBQ can be made lighter without reducing the fun. BBQ doesn't have to always be a guilty pleasure; it can nourish the body as well as the soul.

- **Lean cuts:** Chicken breasts, turkey, or fish
- **Veggie power:** Grilled peppers, zucchini, mushrooms, and even cauliflower steaks
- **Smarter sides:** Instead of dousing sides in mayo, use a vinaigrette. Substitute grilled veggies for baked beans.
- **Portion control:** Focus on the meat, of course, but round out the plate with fresh veggies.

[100]
BBQ STORIES
& LEGENDS

Every BBQ culture has a history and trade secrets passed down through generations. From Texas pitmasters who won't share their brisket technique to Caribbean cooks hiding jerk recipes pre-dating the invention of gas engines, BBQ is full of legends.

Some people say the best BBQ is based, not on taste, but rather on the length of the line to the grill. Others swear that smoke carries memory. One small whiff of hickory can take them back to a childhood summer. As you learn the art of BBQ, you'll join this continuous chain of storytellers, passing along a tradition that's not just food, but history.

[101]
WHY BBQ MAKES YOU
A BETTER MAN

BBQ is fire and patience. It's community and accountability. Over the years, you'll develop respect for time, discover the importance of feeding others before yourself, learn to enjoy life's simple pleasures, and so much more. Ultimately, BBQ sharpens more than your craft—it sharpens your character. Any man can eat, but a pitmaster feeds, hosts, and creates memories that live well after the smoke has cleared.

What BBQ Teaches

- **Discipline:** You can't rush brisket.
- **Generosity:** Good BBQ is meant to be shared.
- **Resilience:** If at first you don't succeed, try, try again!

CONCLUSION: KEEP THE FIRE BURNING

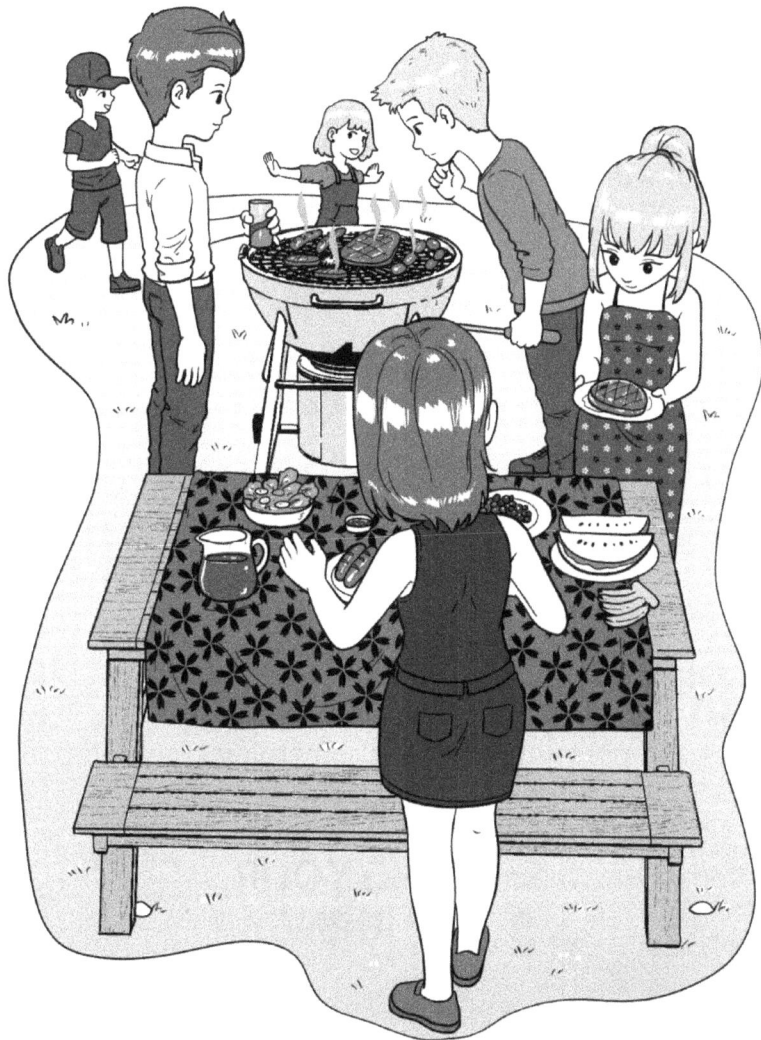

RECAP OF THE JOURNEY

Our 101 essentials have covered everything a pitmaster needs, from the fundamentals of grilling to rubs, sauces, and simmering secrets. We discussed essential gear that makes things easier, cuts of meat that shine on the grill, flavor pairings to enhance a meal, and troubleshooting hacks for when the heat is on.

Additionally, we went beyond food to embrace the lifestyle of BBQ: tailgating setups, hosting from the backyard pit, gift ideas for your BBQ brothers, and grilling traditions from all over the world. As we explored recipes, we built not just flavor but a mindset. You learned about the value of cooking that connects the past with the present, skill with patience, and fire with companionship.

The big takeaway? BBQ isn't just about food. It's about the fire you control, the people you feed, and the stories you create.

ENCOURAGEMENT TO EXPERIMENT

Now, it's your turn. The best BBQ pitmasters didn't get there by following a rigid set of rules. They experimented and failed, then adjusted and tried again. These 101 essentials provide you with a jumping-off point, but feel free to go off script.

Whip up tandoori chicken one week and Texas brisket the next. The fire is your canvas, and the grill is your workshop. Treat each mistake as an opportunity to learn something new, and both your successes and disasters will become epic stories to tell.

SHARING YOUR BBQ JOURNEY

BBQ should never be a silent affair; it's about bringing people together—friends, family, neighbors—and providing more than just a meal. BBQ tantalizes the senses, creating moments around smoke and flame that endure long after the last plate has been cleared.

So share your food, share your knowledge, and share the joy. Post your recipes, swap tips, or welcome a new person at your table. The more you share, the richer your tradition becomes.

At the end of the day, BBQ isn't what you eat, but who you become: a keeper of fire, a host of laughter, and part of a legacy that's as old as man himself. So fire up that grill, and get cooking!

www.ingramcontent.com/pod-product-compliance
Lightning Source LLC
Chambersburg PA
CBHW071701210326
41597CB00017B/2273